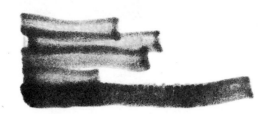

WE CARRIED THE MAT

My faith journey as a primary caregiver
...and how a community made all the difference

KATIE JORDAN

EDITED BY RENEE ANDERSON

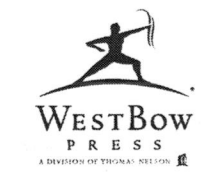

WESTBOW
PRESS
A DIVISION OF THOMAS NELSON

ISBN: 978-1-4497-4956-9 (e)
ISBN: 978-1-4497-4955-2 (sc)
ISBN: 978-1-4497-4954-5 (hc)

Library of Congress Control Number: 2012908327

WestBow Press books may be ordered through booksellers or by contacting:

WestBow Press
A Division of Thomas Nelson
1663 Liberty Drive
Bloomington, IN 47403
www.westbowpress.com
1-(866) 928-1240

Printed in the United States of America

WestBow Press rev. date: 5/16/2012

Dedicated to the "Mat Carriers,"

who selflessly, fervently serve others
in the spirit of Mark 2:1–11

Several days later Jesus returned to Capernaum,
and the news of his arrival spread quickly through the town.
Soon the house where he was staying was so packed with visitors
that there wasn't room for one more person, not even outside the door.
And he preached the word to them.
Four men arrived, carrying a paralyzed man on a mat.
They couldn't get to Jesus through the crowd,
so they dug through the clay roof above his head.
Then they lowered the sick man on his mat, right down in front of Jesus.
Seeing their faith, Jesus said to the paralyzed man,
"My son, your sins are forgiven …
Stand up, take your mat, and go on home, because you are healed.

IN MEMORY OF
Jay Jordan
Bobette Borchardt
Gary Cairns
Ruth Gaines

IN HONOR OF
Ted York

HEARTFELT THANKS AND ACKNOWLEDGMENTS

Pastor Mike Slaughter, for the sermon that led to the writing of this book

Pastor Mike Bowie, for permitting me to use his wit and wisdom freely throughout these writings

The Sowers and Reapers cell group members of Ginghamsburg Church, for their gifts of prayer and physical presence throughout this journey: Pamela and Alan Bailar, Bev Baker, Jeff and the late Bobette Borchardt, Melissa Cairns and the late Gary Cairns, Jim and Linda Dean, Bob and Marilyn Freeman, Rick and the late Ruth Gaines, Reed and Donna Sevitts, Ted and Darla York, and Marcia and Gary Niswonger

Carolyn Slaughter, for making the Night Angels possible

The Night Angels, an elite group of the Ginghamsburg United Methodist (GUM) church family, who gave of themselves for over a year to help put Jay to bed, feed us, sleep over, laugh with us, and unconditionally love us—even though we had never met most of them prior to our need: Jayne and Scott Rowlett, Beth Thoele, Jim and Deb Meyer, Lynn and Chuck Cox, Reed and Donna Sevitts, Kathy Conrad, Cheryl and Dave Jett, Ruth Gaines, Lisa Wright, Tori Peck, and Dave Brown

John Jung, Jay's mentor

Todd Carter, who captured our story through video

Paul Jones, Donnie Reis, and the other talented vocalists and musicians

Ginghamsburg Church Family

The Staff at Good Samaritan Hospital and Samaritan North Rehabilitation Center

The ALS Association's Southern and Central Ohio Chapter

Upper Valley Medical Center Home Health

American Nursing Staff

Hospice of Miami County, Ohio

Hospice of Dayton, Ohio

Dr. Eric Pioro, neurologist at Cleveland Clinic

Dr. Laura Sams, neurologist at the University of Cincinnati, Cincinnati VA, and coordinator of Jay's care

Dr. Thomas Younger, pulmonologist

Dr. Cleanne Cass, hospice physician

Dr. Barb Hill, who managed my health under these extraordinary circumstances

Jay's US Air and Piedmont Families

The Staff of Miami County Jail

The Kentucky Clan, for their countless trips to Ohio: Stanley and Sandy Gulley, Lisa Gulley Hook, Charlie and Francis Bauer, and Audie Jordan

My Family

Mason County High School Class of 1968

Rick Weddle

Catherine Gohrband

Coy Dilhoff

Chris Coughlin, Doctor of Chiropractic

Judie Sturm

Larry and Patti Green

Kim Yardlay

Judy and Jack Fiessinger

"Two Chicks Digging"

Tim, Deanna and Brittany Collins

The OTs, COTAs, PTs, Speech Pathologists, and LMTs who volunteered so Jay could have adaptations, ROM, a communication board, diet information, and massages: Wendy Godwin, Terri Griffin, Donna Fletcher, Melissa Fitzgerald, Summer Dilbone, Laura Bajus, Catherine Gohrband, and Ruth Gaines

Sam Kingery, helicopter pilot extraordinaire

John the Pilot, Piqua Crane & Sidney Fire Department

Cincinnati Veterans Administration Hospital Nurses

Missy Clark

Kelly Labree

The Pallbearers who lifted and carried Jay for the last time: Alan Bailar, Jeff Borchardt, Charles Cox, Rick Gaines, Larry Green, David Jett, Jim Meyer, Scott Rowlett, and Reed Sevitts

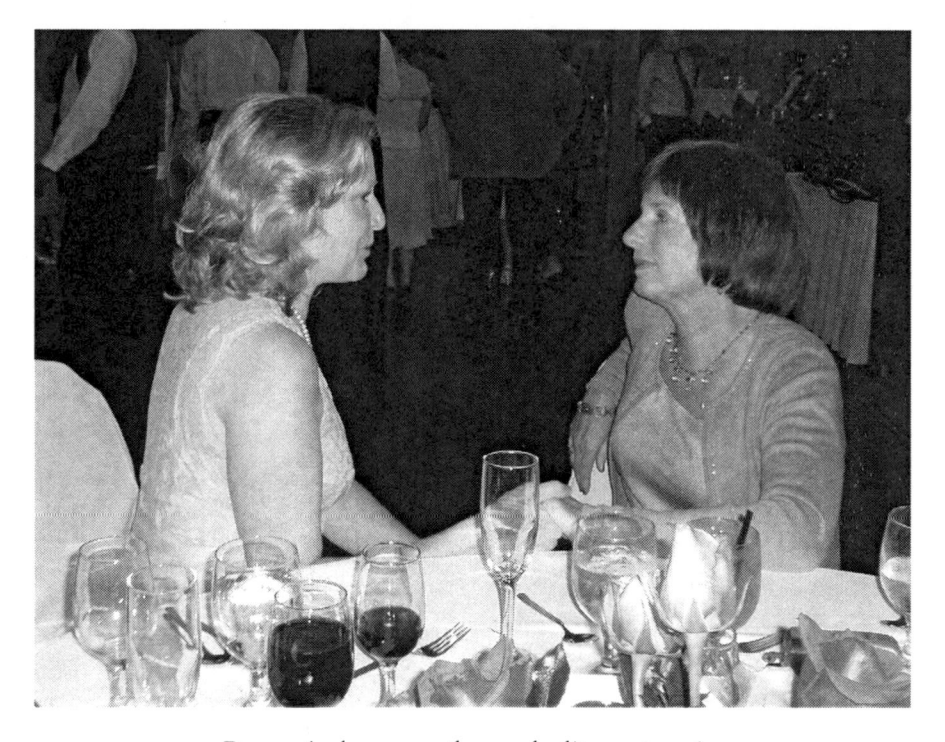

Renee Anderson, author and editor, reassuring
me that God has a plan for my life.

A WORD FROM THE AUTHOR

As a high school student, teachers said I had a natural gift for writing. In college, however, studying to become a physical therapist required me to focus more on mathematics and the sciences. My compositions reflected the cold, hard facts, and I "forgot" how to express feelings and write creatively. Feelings seemed to have no place in my career choice, except in the way I related to patients. By the time I returned to the college classroom years later to earn a master's degree, I felt lost and relied on my husband, Jay, to help revive my lost gift of writing.

Thirty years zipped by. Quite suddenly, in January 2004 (months before Jay's first symptoms), I felt compelled to start keeping a journal. Looking back on those fledgling entries, I recognize now that my decision to begin journaling at that particular time was prophetic.

Writing in that "safe place" reconnected me to my Heavenly Father during the most petulant time of my life. As Jay was losing his battle with amyotrophic lateral sclerosis (ALS; also known as Lou Gehrig's disease), I found solace in being able to write after he was asleep. Even at midnight or later, I found myself groping for the journal and a pen.

At our lowest times, God speaks to us in many ways to keep us encouraged. Often, I found Him speaking to me through others. I can't count the number of times I logged something in my journals that had come from the lips of strangers, friends, mentors, and Bible study teachers. These were bits of light and wisdom I tried to implement in my hectic daily life as Jay's wife and caregiver. Now, I'm so grateful they are recorded as a resource during times of trouble.

In addition, I began recording my prayers, such as, "God, help me put you back in control of my life. I can accomplish tasks better with your help and guidance."

Through journaling, God began to unfold His wisdom. The thoughts began to unfurl and were no longer my own. They seemed to directly flow from the Holy Spirit. When I was so exhausted and confused while taking care of Jay, journaling became an avenue of clarity when all seemed bleak. I could release the day's burdens by writing them down and letting them go. I learned to seek God for wisdom before acting. As Pastor Mike Bowie used to say, "God, move me out of the way."

Keeping a journal of experiences is a wonderful coping mechanism. As you juggle the physical and emotional challenges of being a caregiver or caring supporter of someone who is ill, please consider journaling your thoughts and experiences.

In addition, I hope this book will meet you right where you are and provide encouragement, compassion, affirmation, and hope. You will find God faithful in every step of the way, just as I have. Join Him where He is already at work, and He will equip you to do all that you need to accomplish, just as He led me through my caregiving journey to completion, one step at a time.

May God bless you and keep you in His grace,

Katie

INTRODUCTION

It was a beautiful day in our community just north of Dayton, Ohio. As we strolled the Miami Shores Golf Course, watching our son, Luke, play a round for Troy Christian High School, my husband, Jay, began to complain of a persistent twinge in his right hip.

No big deal, we thought. After all, Jay was fifty-four, a prime age for a few arthritis symptoms to kick in. On our frequent walks together, we had often teased each other about the minor maladies that go hand in hand with the aging process.

But one day shortly thereafter, Jay developed "foot drop"—dragging his right foot and tripping frequently. I worried, but Jay made light of it. "I'm even clumsier than usual!" he quipped.

When severe muscle cramps ensued, I knew Jay was in serious trouble. That is how our two-and-a-half-year journey with ALS began. The disease takes one completely captive before it sets the mind, body, and spirit free.

As a practicing physical therapist, I was initially able to apply my clinical skills and training to help Jay cope with his symptoms as they appeared. Long before we received a confirmed medical diagnosis, I had become my husband's caregiver. His welfare became my sole mission and purpose.

During our last great adventure together, our roles dramatically and suddenly reversed. You see, throughout the course of our two decades as husband and wife, Jay had always been the leader, the comforter, the "cheerer-upper" in our relationship. He was the one who taught me how to let go of my worries, laugh loud and long, and live life abundantly. He took care of me in a way no one ever had or ever will.

In his final months, I had the combined joy and agony of bolstering his emotional welfare and endurance, while providing physical and medical care for him. Every waking moment, I summoned all my strength to be present for him, to buy him a little extra time, to hold onto him for one more day, and finally, to say good-bye.

When I met and married him, Jay had a military background in the air force and served a year in Vietnam, before he went to work with Piedmont Airlines and later, US Air. Throughout his adult life, he embodied the spirit and character of a good and faithful soldier. He intuitively knew how to deal with adversity.

On his worst days, Jay's eyes continued to sparkle with life. In fact, during those trying times, the clarity of God's purpose for Jay's life began to sharpen. He is recorded on video as saying, "If God heals me, wow! I can't imagine what a testimony I will have ... and I'll never shut up! But if God decides that I should go Home to be with Him, the best thing I can do between now and that day is to continue to do His will, not my own."

In truth, Jay delighted everyone with his sense of humor. He had an innate ability to weave confidence and worth into the hearts of others, including mine. In private moments, when no one else was present, I witnessed Jay's struggle with humiliation and depression, as he learned to cope with his terminal condition. Ultimately, however, his spirit found a way to soar high above the indignities of the disease. Even after he could no longer move and had trouble speaking, Jay always managed to exhort friends and strangers alike.

Day in and day out, week by week, month by month ... breath by breath. For two-and-a-half years, we waged war with an enemy that never plays fair. The disease crept upon him like a thief and eventually robbed him of his ability to move, speak, swallow, and breathe. Eldon "Jay" Jordan, whose quick wit and colorful persona had charmed everyone he had ever met, drew his last breath on June 27, 2007, with our dog, Tipper, guarding him closely in her position on his bed. When he had drawn his last breath, Tipper sighed, lay across his body, and went to sleep. She knew his struggle was over, and her job was finished.

I felt finished, too. During those two-and-a-half years, the mirror had gradually begun to reflect an older, wearier me. I heard the exhaustion in my voice and noticed it in my posture. At times, I felt defeated, depleted, destroyed. On that June morning at his graveside, I wondered whether I was burying a piece of myself with Jay.

I remember the moment I had prayed out of sheer desperation for God's help. It was on a day we were being bounced from one doctor's office to another in search of a diagnosis, hoping it *wasn't* ALS. I wondered if God was listening to my prayers, or whether they were bouncing off the ceiling of those medical buildings. So I asked Him for a specific sign—ladybugs—to assure me He was listening and would answer.

God was listening all right, because over the course of the next two years, He sent ladybugs. Lots of ladybugs! They not only came in the "bug" form to remind me on occasion that God was intimately aware of what we faced, but they also appeared in "people" form! In a variety of ways and as special needs arose, people from our community and church walked with us during the toughest journey of our lives. Friends and strangers alike, who had heard of our plight, streamed in and out of our home to help us—sometimes at all hours of the day and night. With them came smiles, encouragement, hope, faith, prayers, and perseverance. Ladybugs to the rescue!

> The Lord hears His people when they call to Him for help.
> He rescues them from all their troubles.
> The Lord is close to the brokenhearted;
> He rescues those who are crushed in spirit.
>
> —Psalm 34:17 NIV

Almost every day, I witnessed tiny miracles and immeasurable love in the face of death. I recorded the experiences, letters, pictures, and descriptions of people who came alongside us in our time of need. They each uniquely blessed us with gifts of time and loving, spirited service.

With the help of Todd Carter from our church and our son, Luke, we recorded a video vignette to share with our church family.

God must have strengthened me during the journey, for I have survived by grace with so much to share. Rich life lessons have been gleaned from the extraordinary challenge and privilege of being Jay's primary caregiver.

In loving Jay through his most challenging journey, I became cognizant that I am not alone as a primary caregiver. Across the United States and worldwide, primary caregivers like me are fighting for the lives of their elderly and other loved ones who suffer the injustices of cancer, ALS, multiple sclerosis, muscular dystrophy, Alzheimer's disease, and myriad of other serious and terminal afflictions. According to the National Family Caregivers Association, there are over fifty million primary caregivers in the United States alone.[1]

They are the ones who rally the call for further research while emptying the bedpan. With God's help, they round up support when it becomes impossible to forge ahead alone. And they do it all with a dose of faith and a healthy sense of humor: God's grace mechanism. Caregivers are a special breed that way. They hang onto tiny comical moments that spawn hope and joy in order to surf the waves of discouragement.

Primary caregivers are society's unsung heroes ——
God's hidden soldiers serving on the battlefield of life and death.
They need affirmation and support from the community.
Creating community awareness and affirming the
caregiver are the dual purposes of this book.

After such exhausting, relentless love in action, the caregiver's efforts are ultimately and tragically rewarded by great loss. When the loved

---

1   National Family Caregivers Association (NFCA) 2009 website. Source: U.S. Department of Health and Services, Informal Caregiving: *Compassion in Action.* Washington, DC: 1998, and National Family Caregivers Association, Random Sample Survey of Family Caregivers, Summer 2000, Unpublished.

one dies, the caregiver is left to pick up the pieces of life, bear the scars, and press forward to find fresh purpose.

Without Jay beside me, life has been a strange new adventure. Everything familiar and comfortable is gone. I feel sort of like Dorothy in Frank Baum's *The Wonderful Wizard of Oz,* after the tornado lifts her house into the sky and sets it down in a strange new land.

Like Dorothy along the proverbial Yellow Brick Road, I've learned to take the journey one step at a time. If I begin to lose my way, I only need to remember the essence of my joy-filled Jay and those who rallied to his side and helped me cope. For now, you see, I have a promise to keep, both to Jay and to God ... and to you, my fellow caregiver.

> "For I know the plans I have made for you," says the Lord.
> "They are plans for good and not for disaster,
> to give you hope and a future."
> —Jeremiah 29:11

This book is a gift of love resulting from a promise I made to Jay several months before he died. During the two-and-a-half years that Jay's body became captive to ALS, he shared his faith and exuberance for life with the servants at his bedside. He shared it through recordings and colorful anecdotes. He chose not to write his story in the eloquent words that he had previously spoken. Rather, in his final months, he wrote it on the hearts of those who cared for him, including mine. Now, the written words of his story—our story—have been entrusted to me.

Jay is most assuredly "somewhere up there," with a wide, satisfied grin on his face, celebrating that the essence of our experience is finally in print. My hope is that you will be encouraged and affirmed, as you seek to help someone you love reach the finish line of life with grace and purpose. I hope that your community will rally about you.

Jay's story is incomplete, until it has fully
encompassed the value of the caregiver.
Through this book, I am passing along Jay's legacy and gift to others,

which was to weave confidence and exhortation into the hearts of others:
namely, caregivers of the seriously and terminally ill.

The title and theme of this book are based on Bible scripture, namely Mark 2:1–11, in which the caregivers of a paralyzed man demonstrated great faith in Christ's healing power. They carried their dying friend on a mat and took him to Jesus, so their friend could be healed.

Seeing the great faith of the paralyzed man's
friends … Jesus healed him.

We Carried the Mat pays tribute to the individuals who sacrificially make a way for their suffering loved one(s) to meet the healing touch of Jesus. Today's "mat carriers" are often overlooked, even as they tenderly care for those suffering. Many of their stories have yet to be written or recognized. In sharing our story, may caregivers find long-deserved affirmation meant to strengthen their confidence and know-how in building a support community. May this book also inspire others to come alongside the primary caregiver to help carry the mat.

God's Promises to the CAREGIVER

I will never leave you nor forsake you.
Joshua 1:5

I will instruct you and teach you in the way you should go;
I will counsel you and watch over you.
Psalm 32:8

I will sustain you and I will rescue you.
Isaiah 46:4

I will strengthen you and help you;
I will uphold you with my righteous right hand.
Isaiah 41:10

I am with you and will watch over you wherever you go.
Genesis 28:15

I have engraved you on the palms of my hands.
Isaiah 49:16

I will walk among you and be your God,
And you will be my people.
Leviticus 26:12

Author's Note: Near the onset of Jay's illness, a friend gave us the Bible verses above and titled them, "God's Promises to Jay." These verses were of extraordinary comfort to both of us—the patient and the caregiver. Hence, I'm including these promises from God, especially as they apply to you, the caregiver, who is reading this book. May you receive comfort and reassurance of God's presence and grace as you cling to the truths of God's promises and carry your loved one to Jesus through faithful care and devotion.

CHAPTER ONE

REFLECTIONS FROM THE HEART: IN A NUTSHELL

The Essence of Jay, Our Life Together, and What Affliction Taught Us

From the first day I met him, Eldon "Jay" Jordan was a silver-tongued wit. His air force nickname, Jay, best suited his charismatic, fun-loving personality and stuck throughout the rest of his life, as did his penchant for dispensing vintage proverbial wisdom. His droll, folksy anecdotes often communicated deeper truths meant to encourage others, including me.

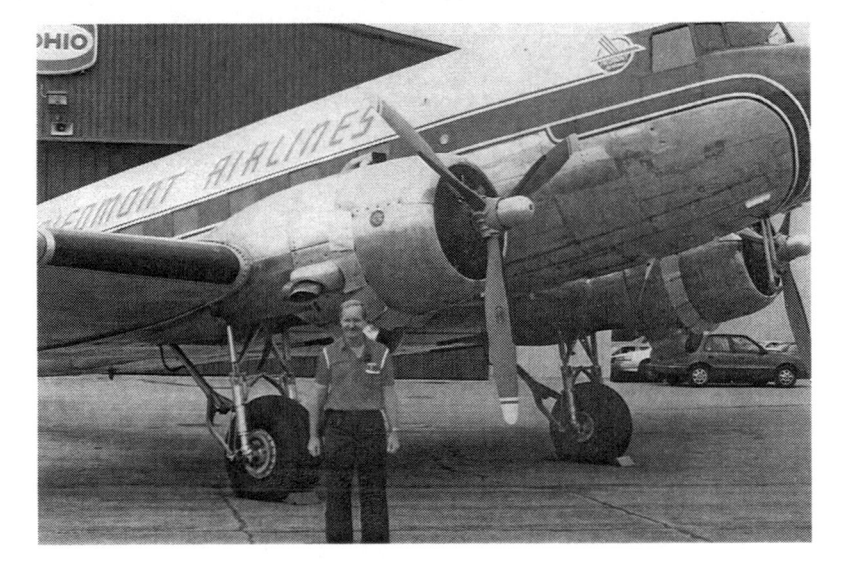

Jay working on the ramp in the early 1980s

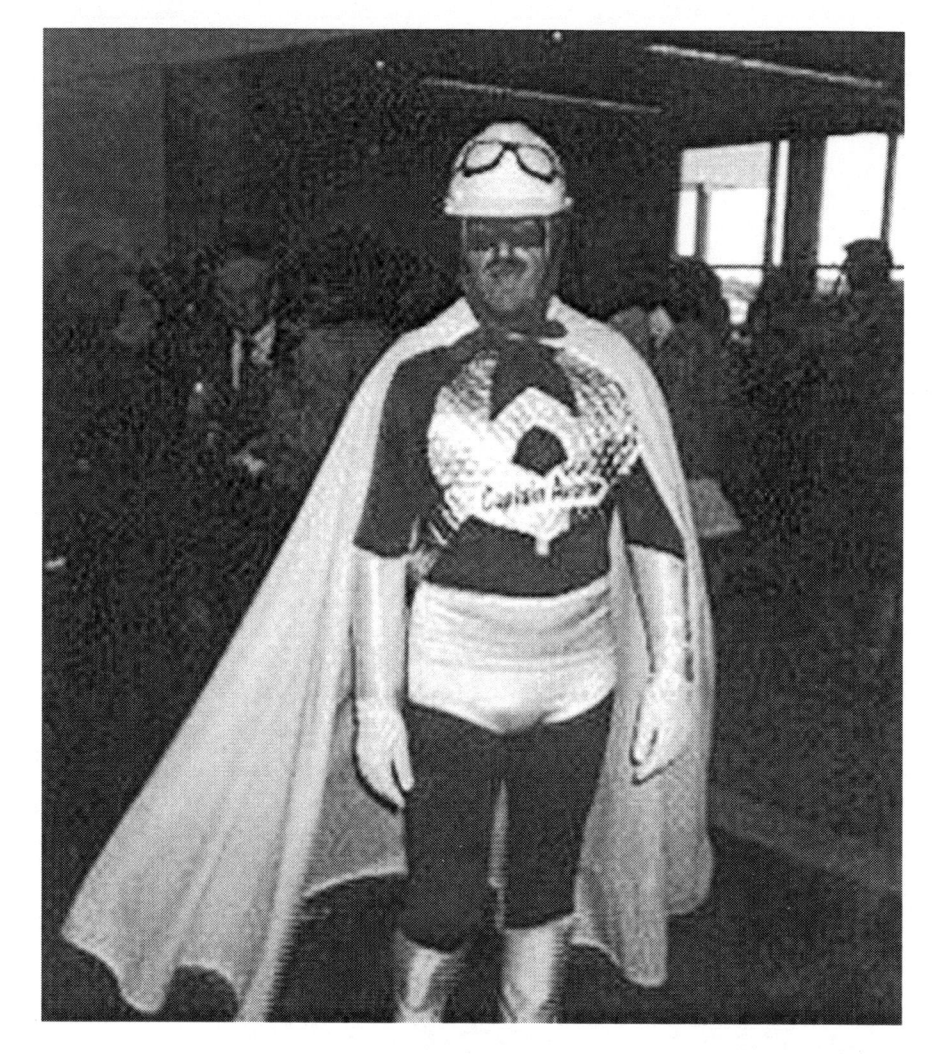

*Jay performing as Captain Aviator at the Dayton
international Airport in the late 1980's.*

Jay and I met when my life was at an all-time low. My husband had left
our home and moved to another town. Our marriage ended, and I was
left with a mortgage and our two small children, Matthew and Sarah.
I had returned to work full time as a physical therapist to support the
three of us.

On Memorial Day weekend of 1985, when Sarah and Matthew were on
a scheduled visit with their father, I had made plans with my coworker,

Sandy, to go out for dinner. She called me later to cancel, because her brother-in-law had unexpectedly come to town. I suggested we just include him in the evening out, as I was a single mother desperate to get out in a social setting with adults!

As it happened, Sandy's brother-in-law was Jay. He was so easy to talk to that I found myself pouring out my life story and all its current confusion. I have no idea what Sandy said that evening. It was all about Jay. I had never met anyone like him!

His childhood stories conjured charming images of rustic Americana. Jay was born at home on February 18, 1950, during a snowstorm in the small town of Flemingsburg, Kentucky. His father, Audie, named him Eldon Wade, because he had read the name in a book and liked it. His parents knew exactly how much he weighed at birth: "about the same as a sack of flour." He grew up without indoor plumbing, and as he said, "I shared my room with a sideboard and a refrigerator—and a dead dog underneath the floor."

Jay described himself as the kind of kid who was ornery enough to break all the eggs under a setting hen. He told me about the time he ran over a chicken with his tricycle when he was three years old ... and the family ate the chicken for supper. Those poor chickens had certainly met their match.

You can imagine dinner the night I met Jay was sparkling with laughter, as the colorful storyteller charmed his audience of two. I also learned that although he considered himself to be an underachiever in school, music inspired him to grow and develop. His school's choral group traveled to England to perform, and that experience changed his life perspective. After high school, Jay entered the air force and served a year in Vietnam. He retired from the military and became an employee of Piedmont's security force.

Whew! Where did the time fly the night I met Sandy and her brother-in-law for dinner? We closed the restaurant, chatting until I think they were ready to kick us out.

The conversation that night extended to every night, as Jay and I chatted by phone between Ohio, where he lived, and Kentucky, where I lived. With his encouragement, I summoned the courage to resolve the issues remaining with the failed marriage. Then I moved and started to rebuild my life as well as my children's lives. Somewhere along the way, Jay and I fell in love, emulating those funny Meg Ryan romance movies, such as *When Harry Met Sally.*

In the months before we married, Jay became my best friend and confidence-weaver. Perhaps because confidence secretly eluded him, he was sensitive to the need in others and sought to bolster them with heartfelt empathy and a hearty dose of comic relief.

Jay and I were married August 1, 1986, and he inherited the responsibilities attached with rearing two stepchildren. Ten months later, Lucas Wade Jordan was born to complete our family.

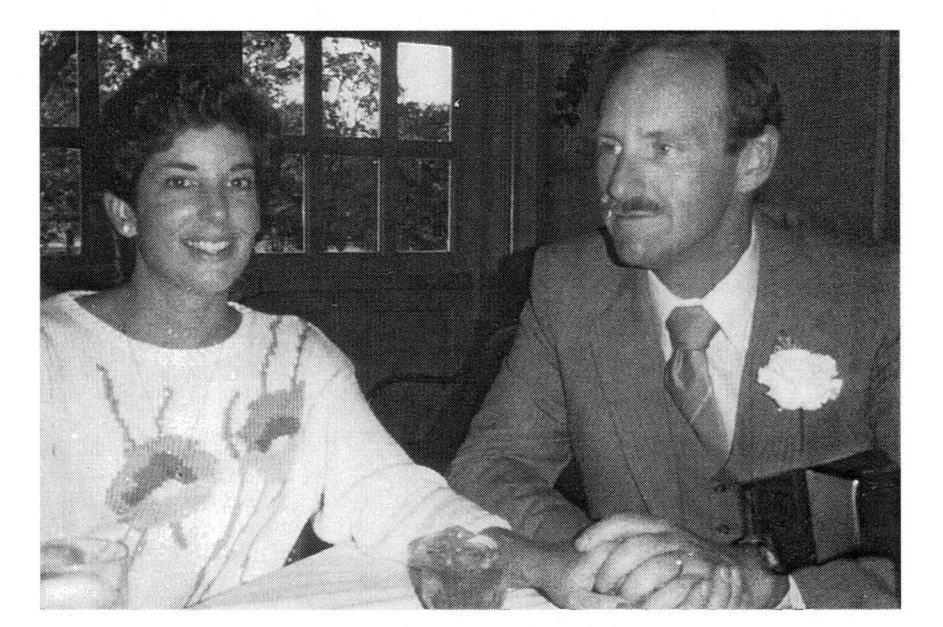

Jay and I on our wedding day

Jay seemed to have an intuitive understanding about how to be a stepfather. He realized it would take time for my two little ones to accept the new man in their mother's life and for trust to take root. I appreciate that Jay never attempted to become their father, because he recognized they already had one. Instead, he was just there for them. Gradually, both children grew to love him and sought him out for needs and emotional support. Beyond that, the kids and I used to joke that Jay was one of the most popular "room mothers" at their school. He was a favorite field trip chaperone with all the children in Sarah's and Matthew's classes.

During the first years of our marriage, we enjoyed a true jet-set lifestyle through the benefit of Jay's employment in the airline industry. Our routine workweeks were punctuated by the spontaneity of flights out of state for specialty dining or a weekend of adventure. Later, with our children, we enjoyed lengthy, fun-filled vacations throughout the United States.

Make no mistake: we didn't have a fairy-tale marriage. There were plenty of highs and lows. But God was right there and brought us through the stormy times, producing an even stronger marriage bond.

Through the years, I marveled at how Jay attracted people. He was hoisted on the shoulders of protégé after protégé. He knew no shortage of friends, and his ability to touch people's hearts with his quick wit and compassion was no stronger than when ALS began to sap his strength.

In the summer of 2004, Luke was about to enter his senior year of high school. Realizing the empty-nest lifestyle was quickly approaching, our focus began to shift toward living as a couple again.

It was an exciting time of planning and dreaming. Just two years prior, Jay had made a career change from employment with US Air to a self-employed owner of a franchise, The Entrepreneur's Source, which perfectly fit his passions. His new role involved talking with people about their "burning bushes"—that is, helping professionals discover their primary interest or passion. Then, he would match them with an appropriate franchise opportunity. Meanwhile, I was soon to attend Capitol University to become a certified life care planner. Together, we looked forward to refreshing our lives with these new vocations, more travel, relocation to a warmer climate, and other "second honeymoon" aspirations.

For years, Jay, a licensed massage therapist, and I, a licensed physical therapist, had known about ALS, as we had worked with ALS patients in our professions. We knew all about the devastating neurodegenerative progression of the disease and how heart-wrenching it was for family members, who helplessly stood by as their loved one declined day after day. We had always declared we would never get *that* disease as though we could will ourselves to avoid it. Oh, how wrong we were.

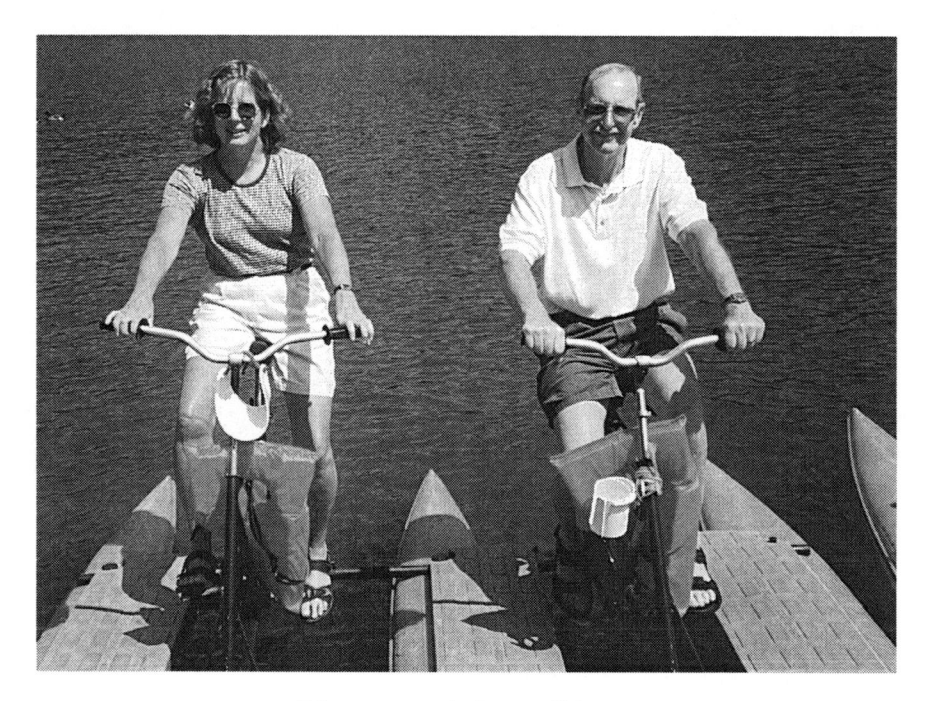

The summer before it all began

It was the fall of 2004 when we began to suspect that Jay *might* have ALS, among other possibilities. Right away, I began researching the symptoms, which prompted moments of sheer panic. Our dreams for the future were under threat of annihilation. Surely this wasn't possible!

Although we never pictured ourselves confronting such an enemy, Jay adopted an attitude of peace from the get-go. He kept saying, "It's going to be all right."

I'd say, "How can it be all right? This is not fair."

Until then, life had always been fair to us. Though I could not fathom the implications of a serious, much less terminal illness, God was with us every step of the way. I eventually developed a spirit of peace, but it was a process. Every time my faith was tested, God would step in with answers to help us around the next bend. In the midst of great adversity, we found ourselves not only surviving the daily challenges but flourishing.

As Jay's neuromuscular debilitation robbed more and more strength from his body, he had lots of time to think about God's purpose in his life. Through wonderful people with whom we worshipped at Ginghamsburg United Methodist Church, Jay realized new, greater purposes God had in mind. For certain, we had been placed way out on a limb, far beyond our comfort zone. Trusting God was the only obvious choice we had. God blessed us with rich opportunities to rise spiritually and mentally above Jay's affliction in our attitudes and outlook.

During his illness, Jay got busy in ministry. He became chairman of the Love Fund, which was established by our church administration to meet the needs of the homeless and poverty-stricken families in the greater Dayton, Ohio, area. As a table facilitator in the Ministry by Strengths class, Jay mentored others. Even as his voice weakened, he became a motivational speaker at the Miami County Jail, among other venues, inspiring others to live out their faith no matter what their life circumstances. Jay was busy fulfilling his fresh new purposes even while his body was busy dying. It was incredible to realize he was touching more lives from a wheelchair than he ever could have as a healthy adult!

We both quit our jobs to take care of the many obstacles we faced. My family came through to help us financially, so we were able to move and build a home designed to accommodate Jay's needs. Because of the gracious financial support of my family, I was later able to go back to school to build a new career for the future.

Ironclad limitations and indignities measured Jay's captive walk through the valley of the shadow of death. While he suffered from an atrophying body and mind, Jay discovered unexpected freedoms. Having already experienced the liberty that comes by serving others, he was now learning the vulnerability of receiving assistance. His humble service to others became allowing friends and strangers alike to serve him. Through his attitude, he nurtured the spirits of servants at his bedside.

Jay was blessed to keep his speech and reasoning until his last months, so he could participate in conversations with friends who stopped in to visit, bring a meal to share, or help with chores. During the course of his illness, he converted several of his friends to his preferred brand of dark beer. They rarely stopped for a visit without the requisite six-pack. As Jay deteriorated, he progressed from tipping the bottle himself to me tipping it, to sipping through a straw. Finally, it was applied with a toothette swab. He had few pleasures left, and we weren't about to take away the beer!

As the result of communicating my desperate need for help, wonderful skilled nurses from our church volunteered their time and energy each night for the last fifteen months of Jay's life. They came at bedtime to help with the rigorous routine of preparing Jay for the night. Our "Night Angels," as Jay dubbed them, were truly the feet and hands of Jesus. They loved us unconditionally, providing spiritual, emotional, and physical support. Their laughter and tears comforted us.

As I reflect on our journey, every time Jay or I cried out to God for help, there was always a "mat carrier" who came alongside us through a phone call, visit, card in the mail, meal, helpful act of service, or a prayer. I will be forever grateful to each individual who stepped up to provide support for this weary caregiver in the cause of providing great care to Jay in his final days and months on Earth.

I felt that God was with us every step of the way, even when we were ready to throw in the towel. He never allowed us to go through a new experience or symptom without also providing the very people who could teach me what I needed to know.

As Jay's primary caregiver, I established a partnership between Jay, our family, and the health-care provider, which continued until his death. At each appointment, I provided a complete list of his physicians, an updated and current medication list, and a notebook to keep track of symptom chronology and appointments. I communicated current needs and asked for help when necessary in developing a plan for Jay's continued care. From the get-go, Jay and I sought out a battery of support services from the ALS Association to the Paralyzed Veterans of America, work contacts, church staff and programs, service clubs, insurance benefits, and friends. Through all the stages of Jay's illness, I learned to be persistent in order to get what his condition demanded. I was reminded often that I had a job; there just wouldn't be any reward to work toward, other than helping Jay to the finish line of his earthly life.

In the first year or so of Jay's illness, I knew how to take care of him because of my training and practice as a physical therapist. In 2006, I began asking for instruction from the nurses and physicians on Jay's case. I learned to give him injections, suction his airway, and deal with the multitude of issues relating to his body slowly losing function and shutting down. If a particular medication didn't work for Jay, I learned to speak up and ask for something else.

The unspeakable loss we experienced encompassed every aspect of our lives. As Jay weakened, we depended on others for assistance, which is greatly appreciated to this day and will be for the rest of my life. But our privacy as a couple was erased in the process. I worried that Luke, who was still in the home at the time of his father's diagnosis, felt he was losing both parents, not just his father.

The intimacy of our marital relationship was lost. I felt robbed of our freedom to make plans for the future and to develop as a couple. I think of all the earthly moments Jay has already missed, I will miss his reactions to and input in each of our family's celebrations and sorrows alike. When Jay could no longer talk, I found myself wanting to probe his mind about what he wanted our future generations to know about him and our life together.

During our twenty years of marriage, Jay's example taught me what a true marriage partnership is. He supported my decisions and stepped into the background when he needed to with the children, so I could shine and devote time to projects and tasks. He assisted me numerous times in my work. He probably deserved the master's degree that I obtained more than I did, since he had a hand in writing most of my papers!

Jay knew when to let me vent and cry. He always knew when to hold me and say nothing. I often wished I could have been as intuitive toward his needs as he had been to mine.

In caring for him, I often felt helpless but never hopeless. It seems that somewhere along this journey, our roles reversed. In my dependence on Jay's support throughout our marriage, we gradually changed roles. He had always been my advocate and best cheerleader; now I was his.

When ALS invaded our lives like a thief, I secretly worried how I would go on without Jay, but I didn't have time to cope with that notion. Jay needed me, and I couldn't break down on him. How surprising then that the Holy Spirit used others, primarily Jay, to patiently and wondrously teach me I would be able to stand alone. As Jay grew weaker, I felt myself growing stronger. Even as tired as I was, it was as if Jay allowed his life force to fill me at his expense. He was passing the torch. Being selfish, I wanted him to hold onto it, but in the final months, he so desperately wanted to let it go.

Although Jay struggled to maintain the semblance of a normal life in his outlook and demeanor, he became increasingly frustrated with his growing number of physical disabilities. After a particularly humiliating experience at a restaurant, he gave me a look I'll never forget. It was so sad and filled with longing. He said, "I just want this to be over."

All I could say at the time was, "I know you do," and then I cried—for him and for me. It would be thirteen months before his prayer to die was answered.

Another time, he asked for a gun. I made light of it, pointing out no one would believe it was suicide, since he had no use of his arms. It was a risk to joke at such a moment, I know. But it worked. In spite of himself, he caught the dark humor and smiled. We connected in a safe place deep in our hearts, where love was strong in the face of fear … beyond his momentary despair.

Balancing the roles of wife and caregiver was my toughest assignment. I had a professional background in physical therapy and routinely dealt with people who required assistance, but I had never used my professional skills on *my husband*.

To know when to be a caregiver and when to be a wife was a tricky walk across a chasm on a very thin tightwire. The caregiver role could easily, and often did, consume me. Jay needed range of motion exercise, massage, balance training, standing time, transfer assistance, and restroom and eating adaptations. At one point, Jay was taking seventy-two pills a day. So you can imagine, after all of these routines, by the time we finished one round, it was time to start all over again.

Everyone—from doctors to specialists to therapists to friends—was eager to give me exercises and tips. Who had time to cuddle? There was no time to "just be." No time for the couple, lovers, friends. Who had time to light candles, sit and listen to music, hold hands on the porch swing in the moonlight, or any of the other special, tender moments we used to share? Life became one big therapy session, with the Grim Reaper looming like a vulture in the room.

One night as I wrote in my journal, I scribbled a weary, desperate prayer that was as honest as I was drained. "God, I miss Jay's bear hugs, the massages, the help, and the real talks. I miss our vacations. I hate the pills, the tubes, the bathroom, and all the confusion in our lives. Too much noise, too many lists, too much equipment, too many sad looks, too little sleep, and too little time to say all I want to say."

When no one else was around, Jay would grow frustrated with himself and with me, as we fumbled through the perfunctory duties of daily hygiene. He clearly felt overwhelmed by all the poking and prodding caregiving required. After all, absolutely nothing was wrong with his mind or his heart. Having to rely completely on me for his physical care and personal hygiene was a degrading invasion of privacy. I knew all that, but the most private of hygiene tasks had to be performed, whether either of us liked it or not. When we were both at our wits' end was the only time my gentle, easygoing Jay would snap at me. At such times, I would retort with indignation, "Do you want me to be your caregiver or your wife?"

There was really no need for Jay to answer. We both knew my question was aimless, angry rhetoric, spawned by these unnatural circumstances that worsened with each passing day. Jay wasn't really angry with me, and I wasn't really angry with him. We were angry at the *disease* for playing dirty, underhanded tricks on our lives; for undermining our relationship; for spoiling the natural balance and joy of our love life; for causing us to become so frustrated that we lashed out at each other in desperation.

Admittedly, being Jay's wife and soul mate took a backseat to being his round-the-clock caregiver. I think Jay's manhood was at stake. He grew increasingly defeated by the knowledge I looked on him as my patient instead of my husband and life partner. The guilt of that plagues me still.

Yet, to this day, I question whether I played the role of caregiver enough? Could I have kept him on his feet longer? Made him more comfortable? Enabled him to be more independent? Kept him one more day? How could I have done more?

That's what caregivers do when overwhelmed: they play the introspective guilt game. As the stress builds, guilt mushrooms like a cloud over a nuclear explosion. Thankfully, we had home health visits and people from church and the community who came into our home to relieve both of us of the angst (more about this in a later chapter).

Everyone who came to help Jay also encouraged me to take mental health breaks—get out for a water aerobics class, a walk, or go shopping with a friend—while Jay kept company with those who came to sit with him, feed him, read to him, or just chat with him. It did us both a world of good.

I don't know how long it took for me to conclude Jay needed his *wife* and a sense of normalcy, not just a therapist robotically going through the motions of patient care. Jay's eyes told me his need, and I certainly needed to get off the treadmill and find a way to relax with my husband while I still had his company. So, I proposed to restore balance into our lives and lead as normal a life as possible under the circumstances.

First, I began to discern what we really needed to accomplish in a given day. I would address the question, What is manageable for us? I began to set aside time free of the extra set of exercises or outside help. There needed to be regular periods of normalcy, in which we could just read, listen to music, watch TV, or talk together. When it was still possible for Jay to enjoy being outside, we would take a drive, just sit on the porch, or plan a casual visit with trusted friends. I remember an outing to a small lake in the country, where we picnicked with our close friends Alan and Pamela Bailar. A change of scenery and the laughter shared was cleansing for both of us, and we felt closely connected again.

Still, there were times that Jay asked me why I stayed with him and did all that I did, day after day, night after night. The question broke my heart. My reply was soft and sure. "Wouldn't you do the same for me if the roles were reversed?" He didn't have to answer. I have no doubt he would have stayed right by me until the end.

Whenever I felt myself becoming the fastidious, frantic caregiver, I took a deep cleansing breath and renewed my purpose to be Jay's wife, in spite of the monumental tasks that had to be done for him. It felt good when we could "just be" together without medical talk. Even when Jay could no longer hold me, to sit on his lap and wrap his arms about me was strangely comforting.

For a weary primary caregiver like me, there was a hidden truth eating away at my spirit. I felt ignored and unappreciated in the public eye. When people greeted us in church or in the community, their eyes were always on Jay, asking how *he* was feeling, encouraging *him*, assuring *him* of their prayers. Despite how grateful I was that Jay was being comforted and affirmed, I began to feel a bit resentful. Didn't those friends think that my son, Luke (who was still at home), and I needed prayer and a little encouraging feedback for the challenges ahead?

Caregivers feel isolated and need validation.

Jay was the one who recognized my secret ache for encouragement. He ended up being the one who affirmed me to others. He talked at length to our cell group about the importance of my role. He talked about my passion in caring for him, and he expressed what I did for him in one word: "advocacy." I cried, because Jay talked from his heart, and I felt the depth of his love.

We both grew in our faith during his final months. At times, faith was all that kept us persevering. But it was enough, because God is enough. ALS is an ugly illness. It was humiliating for Jay and devastating for me, but it taught us complete dependence on God and His timing.

While Jay was sick, I began collecting photographs of everyone who came into our home to help Jay and me cope with ALS. They had become our extended family. I made scrapbooks of pictures and mementos as a celebration of Jay's life, and what a life it was! I am honored to have been his wife, his friend, and his caregiver.

In the years since Jay's passing from this life to his eternal home, I marvel at how Christ has carried me through a labyrinth of uncertainty and loss. He is restoring me to serve Him as an advocate of the primary caregiver.

"Advocacy" is still the word that best describes my life's work and calling. Thanks, Jay, for giving it a name!

CHAPTER TWO

THE BEGINNING OF THE END

The Diagnosis

Jay began experiencing right hip pain in August 2004. By early December, his list of symptoms had grown to include back pain, right foot drop, severe leg cramps, frequent muscle fasciculations, and balance problems.

The protocol during those pensive four months was to take the proverbial two steps forward and three steps back, as we ricocheted from one specialist's office to another. The community of medical professionals found "multilevel neurological involvement" but didn't have a name for it. Deep down, I already knew.

On December 2, Jay told me he was experiencing multiple muscle fasciculations; the movements appeared to scurry like tiny mice just beneath the skin on his arm. We both went to bed with a sense of foreboding. Our professional backgrounds in massage and physical therapy had prompted us to imagine the worst, but we did not discuss our fears with each other. It felt like there was an elephant in the room with us, but we weren't about to acknowledge it to each other.

Later that night, I was awakened by an audible voice that told me, "Jay has ALS." I believe it was the Holy Spirit's way of preparing me for what was to come.

The next morning, I logged onto my computer at work and looked up amyotrophic lateral sclerosis (ALS), or Lou Gehrig's disease. It was all there on one web page after another. Jay had every one of the listed symptoms of this fatal disease. I felt my blood freeze, as fear gripped my heart. But I still couldn't bring myself to discuss it with Jay. I would later discover that Jay had similar concerns and thoughts at that time. Neither of us dared to discuss our fears with our son.

Finally, Luke approached me one evening and asked me what was wrong. He had seen us go from the orthopedic surgeon, to the physiatrist, to the family doctor. Since we hadn't explained why his dad needed to schedule all these medical appointments, Luke felt excluded, abandoned, and scared.

At last, I revealed my suspicion. "I think your dad has ALS—Lou Gehrig's disease," I confided. Luke held me, while I cried with a depth of sorrow that penetrated pockets of my soul that I hadn't known existed.

Jay would later say to our church family, "At the time we told Luke that I probably had ALS, it was a time that he needed to be focusing on his college education, learning about personal relationships, and getting a handle on his future. Unfortunately, he was burdened with the emotional trauma that comes with watching a parent increasingly become an invalid with each passing week. But my son, Luke, said it best when we told him I had ALS. He said, 'Hey Dad, you're in a win-win situation. If you live, you stay here with us. If not, you get to go to Heaven. You can't lose.' I wish I had that kind of insight when I was just seventeen years old."

Luke went immediately to the computer and started researching the disease. We continued our medical rounds, but now, Luke was accompanying us. This was not exactly what we wanted for our son during his senior year of high school, but he was dutiful, loving, and very involved from that moment forward. Sarah and Matt, who were young adults on their own on opposite ends of the country—California and New York—were made aware Jay was seriously ill, but we waited to tell them the details until we had a confirmed diagnosis.

Although Jay was referred to more specialists, we had to wait until December 22 and January 31 for his appointments with them. On December 22, the doctor observed the fasciculations firsthand. Based on the tests, she concluded that these symptoms were (unfortunately) not caused by pinched nerves or narrowing of the joint spaces in the spine. We saw the grave concern in her facial expression.

Jay remained hesitant to share all the details of his symptoms with Sarah, Matt, and Luke, but at least we had "removed the elephant in our living room." In other words, we didn't tiptoe around the subject any more and were able to talk about it—to some degree. Jay and I both knew in our hearts what the definitive diagnosis would be, even though we couldn't wrap our minds around the gravity of it. We seemed to live on adrenaline.

I felt compelled to get organized and decided to record contact information that might be of help to us during Jay's illness. I picked up my journal to begin my list. Before I could start recording the names of medical staff, specialists, institutions, and organizations that might help us, my eye was taken back to my first entry, which was written several years before we realized Jay was sick. How prophetic that I wrote the following:

> I have had this thought for several days, and I feel the Holy Spirit is pushing me to record my thoughts. I have such a difficult time remembering God's many blessings. When they happen, I feel that they will stay with me, but they don't. I want to see how God is working in my life and be able to share with others.

The first time we heard a doctor say, "possibly ALS," or, "possibly Lou Gehrig's disease," was on January 3, 2005.

Like a thriller movie or suspense novel, our sense of dread had intensified.

But our experience was not fiction. We couldn't wake up or shake off our concerns. This was real. We were living our worst nightmare.

I began anticipating how our lives were going to change. The security of life had already been ripped away from us. That still small voice of God's presence reminded me it was best that I could not foresee the full measure of what was to come. He had placed us in a "grace bubble" of care that carried and protected our minds and hearts as we faced a roller coaster of emotions and a battery of further medical tests.

A local neurologist ordered blood work to rule out diseases that bore similarities to ALS. Jay had already endured a staggering number of tests, but more tests were required to measure muscle enzymes, one to rule out Lyme disease, and one to measure a multitude of thyroid/hormone functions. A follow-up appointment was scheduled to review and discuss test results.

If all were normal, he suggested a spinal tap and/or a muscle biopsy would be in order. He planned for an EMG on January 21, which would be compared to the EMG that was performed on November 9, 2004. An MRI was ordered for the neck, along with blood work.

On January 17, 2005, we went for a second opinion. At this time, I provided a chronology of symptoms as recorded in my journal. It was felt that ALS was a possibility. He resisted delivering that diagnosis due to its finality. I appreciated his grasping at straws, because it gave me just a little more time to hope for a miracle. The doctor stated some treatable cancers mimic ALS, and he recommended we go to Cleveland Clinic. He would ask his contacts there to facilitate Jay's case. More tests were ordered: another MRI, blood work, and a bone and body scan.

When will this nightmare ever end? I prayed.
But I knew it was just beginning.

When we finally arrived for the conclusive report in January, we held our breath. After several hours of being poked and prodded with needles, Jay was ready for answers. The doctor started to leave the room. As he backed out, he very clinically informed us the tests were conclusive. Jay had ALS. Terminal.

The evil invader of Jay's nervous system had a name at last.

We were left alone to deal with the news. Although we had suspected this for months, there were no words for the fullness of our grief in those first moments of this conclusive knowledge. The only thing to do was hold each other, cry, and try to gather our wits.

As we passed the receptionist's desk on our way to the exit, I asked about scheduling a return appointment. "There's no need to schedule another appointment," the receptionist replied, her eyes avoiding mine. "I'm sorry, but there is nothing more we can do for your husband."

So this is what it's like to receive a death sentence, *I thought.*

CHAPTER THREE

ADJUSTING OUR LIFESTYLE AND MIND-SET

How Staying Busy Helped Us Cope

No more ifs and hypotheticals. At last, the medical world finally confirmed what we had suspected all along. Now what?

As we drove away from the neurologist's office, we faced a barrage of challenges. How were we going to pay the bills since Jay couldn't work, and I would need to quit my job to take care of him? How long did we have until Jay would lose his mobility entirely? How would I be able to lift him? Where would we turn for assistance?

The list of questions racing through my head and heart were infinite. For every question answered, several new ones popped up.

Accommodating a terminal prognosis meant everything about our lifestyle needed to change in every way. We were instantly saying good-bye to our home, our security, our innocence as a family, the way our friends looked at us, the way we related to each other. Everything. This disease was pillaging our lives and taking us hostage. Life became a race against the clock to make as many adjustments as we could while Jay still had use of his body.

After hearing the neurologist's confirmation of our worst fears, we went out to lunch, which we were barely able to touch. Through our tears, we immediately started to plan. I began to make a list of things we needed to do. Thoughts and ideas were coming faster than we could write them down.

- modify our multilevel, sprawling house or move.

- resign from my job or find a job in physical therapy I could handle in addition to taking care of Jay

- Jay resign from new business venture

- communicate diagnosis with family, pastor, and our church cell group

- address the US Department of Labor's Family and Medical Leave provision and other government resources

- see an attorney to draw up advance directives and wills

- make dietary changes that might help enrich and prolong Jay's quality of life

- locate support service agencies, support groups, home health equipment

I stopped writing and closed my eyes in disbelief. Any one of these items on our list could be overwhelming in itself. Put them all together, and it was a full-blown mission impossible. Yet, I had no choice. I had to keep pressing forward to try to find solutions. Now I was the caregiver of my precious, terminally ill husband. I picked up the pen and began to add to the list with new resolve, as our ideas tumbled forth.

Staying busy helped us cope.

Before we did anything else, Jay and I decided to meet with a known prayer warrior, Sue Nilson Kibbey, the executive pastor of Ginghamsburg Methodist Church. Pastor Sue had designed and written many of the curriculums for courses we had attended and taught, such as "Forgive for Good," and "Now, Discover Your Strengths." Her low-key, wise, abiding nature and gift of healing made her an approachable confidante as we sought spiritual guidance.

"What is your greatest fear?" she asked Jay.

Jay didn't hesitate in his reply. "Not being able to serve others anymore," he replied.

I sat quietly, marveling at Jay's answer. I resisted piping up with a comeback remark like, "What? My greatest fear is Jay is going to die."

That's when Pastor Sue said steadily, "Jay, you will best serve others by allowing them to serve you."

Then she prayed with us, and we cried. I think our meeting helped Jay see he could still be useful in exhorting others as they served his physical needs. We left Pastor Sue's office encouraged. In the next few days and weeks, we only shared the news with those closest to us. Our church cell group of about sixteen members prayed with us and came alongside us. Jay told them he struggled with allowing others to serve him. At the same time, he realized he would be stealing their blessings. This act would be his gift to them.

In those first weeks and months of 2005, most of our circle of influence was unaware of Jay's problem. However, occasionally, Jay would spring the news on a passerby on the street. Once, a young lady saw Jay using his cane. Thinking he had sprained his ankle or stubbed his toe, she inquired innocently, "So what happened to you?"

Jay answered, "I've got ALS. But not to worry—dying will fix it." And he kept walking. My heart went out to that poor, bewildered girl. It seemed Jay was determined to take his illness in stride, even joke as much as possible, but this was ridiculous! She clearly was kicking herself for opening mouth and inserting foot.

"Jay!" I reprimanded. "You can't do that to people."

Addressing our bullet points …

Aside from keeping my husband's mischievous humor in check as much as possible, the priority requiring our immediate attention was to determine what sort of housing would best accommodate Jay's growing needs. We already knew that without major modifications, our two-story house with a full basement on Fox Run in our community of Troy, Ohio, would rapidly become a liability. Our bedroom and bath were upstairs. A step-down into family room and the sunroom would complicate Jay's mobility in the house. In addition, his office was located in the basement.

Even with these obstacles, we decided to consider modifying our house to assist with Jay's mobility. His office could be moved upstairs, and perhaps our bedroom and bath could be relocated onto the main level. Our close friends, who had construction modification experience, assessed the feasibility of adding a master bath and bedroom on the first floor. That would still leave us with a step-down into the family room, out of the house, and into the sunroom. Our brother-in-law, Neil, built a platform with rails into the garage to address an immediate need.

Fortunately, prior to Jay's diagnosis, we had already considered downsizing to a smaller house when Luke left for college. Luke had been accepted at Wright State University in Dayton and would begin classes in the fall. With the ALS diagnosis confirmed, the move would have to be sooner rather than later.

With Jay already dependent on a walker, we realized we would need to relocate to a fully handicapped-accessible dwelling as soon as possible. I knew and loved every inch of our comfortable, sprawling home, where our family laughed and loved. Under the circumstances, there was no time for waxing sentimental over the memories. Relocating was inevitable. But to where?

Jay launched an exhaustive search for ranch-style houses listed for sale in the area that would accommodate a wheelchair and allow modifications to the bath. Nothing on the market met those requirements.

Jay's inability to work meant our financial picture was bleak. It was financially impractical to build a new house with custom features to accommodate home health equipment and wheelchairs. But my parents made it possible for us to purchase a lot and build a fully handicapped-accessible home in a new neighborhood development nearby. What a tremendous blessing! The phenomenal expenses involved with medical care financially ruin so many families facing terminal illness. My parents blessed us in a beautiful way that would sustain us through many uncertain times ahead.

As our plans for relocation solidified, we simultaneously worked on a barrage of other projects. Because of Jay's term in the air force, he was able to obtain Americans with Disabilities Act (ADA) building guidelines through the Veterans Administration. Using online search engines, we learned of other resources that might help us and requested them. We quickly became scholars on handicapped accessibility and related subjects.

I contacted the Central and Southern Ohio Chapter of ALS on February 3, 2005. Unlike organizations providing support services and guidance to individuals with Alzheimer's disease, heart disease, cancer, and other serious and terminal diseases, we discovered the National ALS Association is a comparatively fledgling organization. Yet it is the only agency that solely represents the interests of individuals with ALS and their families. Although Lou Gehrig was diagnosed in 1939, the medical community remains baffled by what the National Institutes of Health has designated, "an orphan disease," meaning less than two hundred thousand individuals have been diagnosed with the disease. Very little has been learned about its cause, and because there is little financial incentive for pharmaceutical companies, few effective treatments have been developed. There is still no known cure.

We found a Greater Dayton area support group and began attending meetings. There, we learned that the incidence ratio of ALS is six to eight in every one hundred thousand Ohioans. However, in our area, the average was much higher at that time, with 425 diagnosed with ALS.

I was directed to the ALS loan closet in South Dayton, where we borrowed a transport wheelchair, a cane, and a walker. I registered for the informational monthly newsletter, through which we could obtain practical guidance. We met with Pinky Dressman, the ALS's Dayton area patient services coordinator, who provided further orientation. It was as if we had joined a "club" and were undergoing freshman initiation. Jay was now known as a PALS (person with ALS), and I was dubbed a CALS (caregiver of a PALS). She recommended keeping a relationship with our family doctor for symptom management and home health referrals.

Pitfalls ensued as we discussed Jay's diagnosis with our family doctor, who, under the circumstances, refused his case. After going from physician to physician, we eventually located Dr. Laura Sams in Cincinnati, who was more than willing to work with Jay and coordinate a plethora of issues related to his care. (Since Jay's death, Dr. Sams has continued to correspond with me, and I am forever grateful for her compassion and expertise.)

We were disappointed (but not surprised) to learn Jay would not be eligible for Medicare until five months after his application had been processed. At this writing, that policy has changed. With diagnosis, Medicare can now be received immediately.

As we waited for Medicare benefits to start, we researched whether Jay would be a good candidate for clinical trials and if the expensive drugs would slow the disease and enhance his life expectancy. We sadly discovered Jay's life expectancy might be enhanced by only an additional three months, even if his body would respond to the expensive experimental drugs.

Although Jay was resistant to schedule a meeting with our attorney,

Bill McGraw, to draw up advance directives and wills, he ultimately made the call. However, he didn't share his diagnosis with Bill. During our meeting, when Jay excused himself to the restroom, Bill observed Jay dragging his foot and looked at me with alarm. I told him Jay had been diagnosed with ALS, and the prognosis was terminal. Later, Bill, a devout Christian, prayed with us.

As Jay led the charge on research, I worked on his physical therapy and diet regimens. On Valentine's Day, I watched Jay walk out of Ruby Tuesday following our meal. Observing the muscle tightness in his thighs, I encouraged him to do some simple stretches on the floor at home. After he did all he was physically capable of doing on his own, my PT experience took over. I stretched his hamstrings and helped him with a "shotgun" procedure that would aid in his flexibility. Once he stood up, he practiced walking laps around the downstairs of our home. His gait was much improved. Jay grinned thankfully and remarked, "That workout is the best Valentine's present you could have given me!"

The next morning, he awoke rather surprised he had slept all night for the first time in months. We both stretched before getting out of bed. I helped to stretch his hamstrings further. I once again noticed abdominal fasciculations and observed atrophy in his buttocks. I resolved to repeat the exercises each morning as a daily act of love for Jay and worship to God.

During the same period, our diet completely changed to organic foods. My sister, Betsy referred to our eating habits as, "the nuts and twigs diet." We discarded all plastic, stopped buying canned goods, and researched mercury poisoning. I detoxified every morsel of food before it ever touched our lips. By spring, I had lost eleven pounds and felt much healthier. Reflecting now, I can only imagine those dietary changes enhanced my endurance for the months and years of caregiving ahead.

In the process of juggling so many of life's variables relating to Jay's fresh diagnosis, keeping my wits intact was severely tested. There were times when my thoughts swirled so fast and furiously that I'm not sure "coping well" was in the cards. Trying to sleep at night had become a fitful activity at best. There were so many issues to deal with at once that I wasn't sure where I was half the time.

Focusing on my job at Good Samaritan Hospital in Dayton was becoming almost impossible. One day that spring, I walked down the main corridor of the hospital, lost in thought. It was beginning to hit me that Jay and I had reversed roles. Jay had always been my advocate and cheerleader. Now I was his. *Would I be able to keep up his spirits? Would I be able to physically manage the demands of caregiving? Would we financially survive this trial? Would I be able to let him go when the time came? How would I live without him?* Questions tumbled in my mind like clothes in a dryer.

Just ahead of me in the corridor was a couple who had stopped in their tracks, appearing quite confused. Knowing the hospital's layout like the back of my hand, I offered to point them in the right direction. The couple thanked me and started toward their destination. Then, the gentleman paused and turned back. With a cheesy grin on his face, he asked, "So, are you the CEO of this hospital?"

Laughing, I replied, "No, I'm just someone who looks for lost people."

The gentleman's eyes softened. "That's what Jesus was sent to earth to do," he said. He rejoined his wife, and they disappeared around the corner.

That brief exchange might have taken a minute at most, but it was just what was needed to bolster my faith. What a gentle reminder that God cared about what I was experiencing. Though I couldn't predict the future, or how I would cope with it, my spirit was assured that God would see me through this sorrowful journey one step at a time.

A sense swept over me that Jay's and my experience with death and dying would somehow be purposeful. If we took Jesus by the hand, He would show us the way through our maze of questions and concerns.

As I proceeded down that hospital corridor, the heavy burden I was carrying lifted. An aura of peace quieted my mind in submission to the Holy Spirit's presence.

That couple will never know how much their need
of direction helped me to find mine.

By spring 2005, Jay had resigned his job, and it was only a matter of time before I followed suit in order to take care of him full time. Our lives had changed entirely, and our course had been established in the weeks since Jay's diagnosis. I can clearly see how God was making a way for us, as we entered the valley of the shadow of death. During that chaotic time, His grace was upon us, providing the wherewithal to cope with Jay's diagnosis by keeping us busy. Very busy!

CHAPTER FOUR

MUSICAL HOUSES

Caregiving While Packing and Moving—Twice!

Only a few people knew about Jay's diagnosis in those first uncertain weeks. However, we gradually informed our family members and friends in our church cell group, a small, intimate bunch known as the Sowers and Reapers. These friends, who regularly met for social interaction and Bible study, became very supportive of us during the course of Jay's illness. Among the myriad ways they demonstrated support was through their prayers and actions that helped us relocate twice!

When we put our 4,500-square-foot, multilevel house on the market, it took only sixteen days to sell at the full asking price! That quick sale was a true victory but presented another challenge: to find and move into a rental home in our community by the closing date of July 12, 2005. We asked our church friends in our Bible study to pray with us as we searched.

For whatever reason, while I was anxious we wouldn't make the deadline, Jay had a peace about the situation. He kept saying, "We'll have a place to go by Friday, July 1."

At 5 p.m. that Friday, just as Jay had predicted, we not only had a rental home lined up, but it was offered to us on good faith, without any written lease agreement or signature. It was a one-story rental on Huntington Drive in our community of Troy, Ohio. We had quite a challenge ahead of us: to downsize from our sprawling house filled with sixteen years of collectibles in order to move into a small, ranch-style home in just a matter of days!

Jay and I concluded that many of our belongings were "just stuff" we didn't truly need. Since he couldn't help me pack, Jay set out to enlist reinforcements. He phoned our long-time Fox Run neighbors, who came out in droves to help us. There were people packing everywhere. Storage pods were delivered and filled. An auctioneer came to pick up things to be sold. In addition, we scheduled several inspections and made the recommended repairs, which went along with the sale of our house. As Jay said, "It was a zoo, but God was at work."

On July 9 and 10, we moved into our rental home, where we lived reasonably comfortably, while our handicapped-friendly house construction began. We certainly couldn't have made this dramatic transition without our community of friends.

Building *any* house under the best of circumstances can be stressful, but doing so while coping with Jay's progressive illness added many challenges. There was a time crunch involved. Jay was losing mobility, although he insisted on operating the riding lawn mower at our rental home with a little boost from me. Implementing the special features necessary to accommodate Jay's disabilities added extra anxiety and frustration to the construction process. Perhaps it didn't help that the builder had never previously built a handicapped-accessible home.

By the time we finally broke ground, Jay required a manual wheelchair for transportation outside the house. For him to access the construction site, a wheelchair-accessible pathway was needed so we could cross the heavily rutted, muddy, and sometimes steep areas. Never mind the construction debris that increased our difficulties in navigating Jay's wheelchair from the car into the house.

Looking back, we would have appreciated even a plywood path so that Jay could inspect progress on a regular basis with me. After all, he was the one who needed to be able to determine particulars, such as the height and position of light switches, walls, doorways, and other modifications. Just imagine how grateful we were when a dear couple, Jack and Judy Fiessinger, made us a temporary ramp so that Jay could get on and off the property!

Most of the time, however, Jay waited in the car, while I took digital pictures of the construction progress to show him. From those pictures and my descriptions, we would formulate questions and comments to address with the builder. Then, Jay would e-mail and/or call the builder the next day.

Hindsight is still the best teacher. Perhaps we should have enlisted a knowledgeable friend to monitor progress regularly. It would have saved a lot of starting over on various aspects and details of the house construction. However, through our trial-and-error method, we developed a how-to list for others in our situation. Our article, "Helpful Hints: Home Modification," was published in the Central and Southern Ohio ALS newsletter! (This information can be found in the appendix.)

Preparing Jay for outings was a maneuver of monumental proportions, but we managed to direct our house construction by frequently inspect the progress. We often found ourselves redirecting the workers.

While discussing paint colors with Desi, our site superintendent wanted to know how Jay had become such a strong Christian. Jay shared his story about finding God's purpose and joy in living every day fully for Christ, despite the circumstances. Desi eventually said, "I can see the light of Jesus showing through your eyes."

He asked Jay to speak at his church. Jay and I were not only building a house of mortar and brick. The indwelling Holy Spirit was becoming strong in Jay, who, despite his weakness, had become a lighthouse of inspiration. God was teaching us our suffering was not even about us but about others' seeing God's grace and power working through our weakness.

Since I know it is all for Christ's good,
I am quite content with my weaknesses
and with insults, hardships, persecutions, and calamities.
For when I am weak, then I am strong.
—2 Corinthians 12:10

CHAPTER FIVE

JAY'S GREAT EXPECTATIONS

A Healing Perspective

Life in my hands is a mess; in God's hands, it is a message.
—Mike Bowie, Associate Pastor
Ginghamsburg United Methodist Church, Troy, Ohio

By late summer of 2005, Jay's body had declined to a more dependent stage. He began wearing braces to help support his legs and used a walker. Already, he required far more care than I could manage without resigning my job. Although we were aware Jay's illness would likely financially strap us, I took a leap of faith and resigned. My hope was that somehow we could stay financially afloat for however long Jay needed me. Since Medicare benefits had not yet begun, and as our house construction continued, I asked a few close friends to pray with us that God would supply our financial needs.

Keep on asking, and you will be given what you ask for.
Keep on looking, and you will find.
Keep on knocking, and the door will be opened.
—Matthew 7:7

On August 5, 2005, the director of human resources of Good Samaritan Hospital, my former employer, phoned to inform me I would receive 70 percent pay and health-care benefits for a full six months beyond my date of resignation! This was nothing short of a miracle and a direct answer to our prayers! We could breathe easier in the knowledge we would be financially sustained through February 2006.

Of course, there were plenty of other matters about which to worry. As a nurturer, imagining worst case scenarios was one of my specialties. Jay labeled me a pessimist. I reminded him that someone had to be realistic. Someone had to stay on top of Jay's medical team to make sure his meds were adjusted when necessary. Someone had to monitor the visitors who came and went from our home. Someone had to perform the lifting and the transfers for outings. Someone had to plan the future of Jay's care. Someone had to address the unpleasant issues, like making sure we had enough insurance, setting up meetings with attorneys to develop wills, and with ministers and funeral directors. Like it or not, that someone was I: the primary caregiver.

While I donned a hard-hat attitude for our fight with terminal disease, Jay adopted a childlike faith. As he counseled with mentor John Jung and other leaders in our church, a peace that passes all understanding swept through him that could not be humanly explained. Everyone who came to the house to visit could attest to his spiritual freedom.

Jay refused to let ALS steal the joy he found in his faith. He readily became content to accept his destiny, whether God chose to heal him or take him home to Heaven. Even as he battled frustration with his loss of physical independence, the grace of God empowered Jay to continue serving others. If Jay was destined to die, he was determined to go out with an audience hanging on every word!

On August 7, 2005, he was invited to be the speaker at our church's Healing Service. Jay moved forward slowly on his walker and stood with effort at the podium to speak about his destiny. The following excerpt is from his address to the crowd that day:

> The one thing I am learning as I go through this ordeal is that it is not so important about being physically healed but gaining a closer relationship with God. It is the spiritual healing where

we have the greatest need. He is telling me to reach out and help others who are hurting, who are feeling lost, alone, and afraid. He is giving me numerous opportunities to teach people about this particular illness, how they can help, and how they, in turn, can receive His blessing. He is also healing me in ways that I didn't even realize that I was broken.

I didn't realize how messed up I am! My arrogance of always wanting to do everything on my own and doing it my way has been removed. I still want to, but the ability to do so is gone. My level of impatience with others who are slow to do things or choose to do them differently than I do is being sorely tried, and I am slowly but surely learning this is not the way to live and treat others.

While reading a daily devotional recently, I came across one of those aha moments. Some of you may have seen this if you get the *Purpose-Driven Life Daily Devotional.* The promise was that troubles, confusion, knock-downs-drag-outs are to be expected in a life of faith. They are not just something to suck up and endure, but are the release of God's power in our lives. We encounter deathlike experiences so that Christ's lifelike nature may be clearly seen in us, despite what is happening. It's not just endurance training but God's strategy for ministry through us. His strategy is His power and strength through our weakness. This doesn't just happen to some Christians; it happens to all of us if we want to be effective in our faith.

Whatever the amount of time the Lord wants me to stay here, my prayer is to be able to glorify God's strength through my weakness. I know I have plenty of weakness, and God has more power than I can begin to understand. I believe we could make a pretty good team if I don't get in His way and mess it up.

The sheer honesty and vulnerability of Jay's message was spellbinding. His ability to spin wit and wisdom endeared him to everyone. He had become a role model to a following of awe-inspired supporters.

Not long after the Healing Service, we had our friends Jeff and Bobette Borchardt over for pizza. Bobette had been diagnosed with terminal lung cancer, so a get-together was in order. You might think it would be a somber occasion, but we spent a lot of time laughing and snapping silly photographs. Jay elected to wear Bobette's chemo wig, while she favored a pretty blue scarf. Considering his receding hairline, Jay concluded that Bobette's wig made a big improvement. Laughter ruled, despite the circumstances. Bobette often noted that get-togethers like this one were like a "big hug" to her soul, and we all agreed.

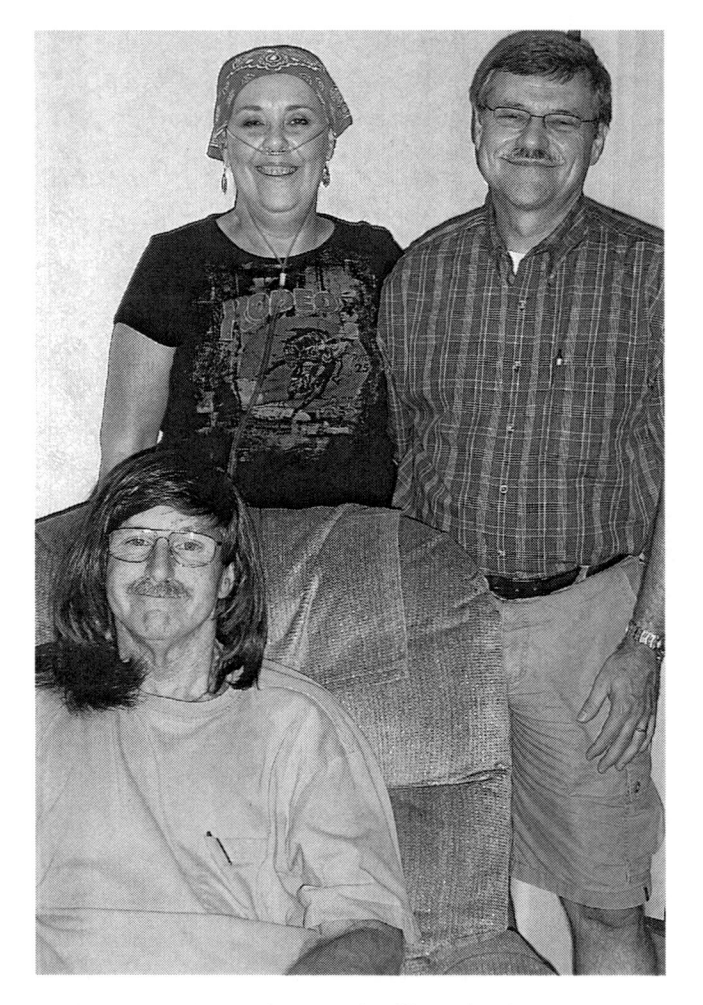

Jay, Bobette and Jeff Borchardt

What happened later that evening revealed a facet of God's grace to Jay and Bobette I had never before witnessed. Bobette's husband and I sat back in amazement, as the two friends connected in deep philosophical conversation about their terminal diagnoses and death. Although their bodies were dying, Jay's and Bobette's souls burst with vitality and life. Already, they seemed to be in Heavenly places only they could understand. They shared a common vantage point, as they perched on the precipice of death.

I recognized that Jay was able to be much more straightforward with Bobette regarding the progression of his illness than with anyone else, even me. And why not? They clearly shared a common bond beyond the obvious challenges of their respective illnesses. Like two wide-eyed children playing in a spiritual sandbox, they spoke with anticipation and peace about meeting their Abba Father face to face.

Don't be troubled.

> You trust God, now trust in me.
> There are many rooms in my Father's home,
> And I am going to prepare a place for you.
> If this were not so, I would tell you plainly.
> When everything is ready, I will come and get you,
> so that you will always be with me where I am.
> —John 14:1–4

That night, I pondered how emotionally detached my husband had become from me as he prepared for his journey to Heaven. Yet, it was only natural, for we had been intimately traveling the same road together for years. Now we were approaching a fork in our journey's path. My journey was to remain the earthly one, while his path was leading him to his eternal home.

In observing this new, strange development in my husband's behavior, I simultaneously felt polar opposite emotions: joy and melancholy. My heart felt torn in half. As Jeff and I sat on the sidelines of their forthright conversation, peppered with hope and faith in their eternal destination, there was nothing to do but be present for our Heaven-bound spouses and reserve our tears for ourselves. Grief had only just begun for those of us who were being left behind.

> When all my plans and hopes are fading like a shadow,
> When all my dreams lie crumbled at my feet,
> I will look up and know the night will bring tomorrow,
> And that my Lord will bring me what I need.
> —Gloria Gaither

That fall, Jay continued praying for healing, believing he really could be healed if it was God's will. I also prayed incessantly for Jay's healing, but I never felt the peace that God would do so. I would lie in bed at night, wide-awake, wondering if I lacked faith. Jay still believed it could happen. Why couldn't I?

One night, I had a dream that Jay was walking around with his braces on, but he was walking normally, upright, without his walker. *What does this mean?* I wondered. *Is this an indication of a healing? Am I glimpsing what Jay will be like in Heaven?*

I think those restless dreams represented my own coming to terms with the unknown. It was a constant internal battle to leave my concerns in God's care. In a way that only a caregiver can understand, I began to learn to live in the moment, and to live in the moment as abundantly as possible. If I needed help lifting Jay in that moment, that is how I prayed: "Dear Lord, strengthen my hands and back for this next lift." And once I had successfully lifted Jay, I'd pray, "Now help me safely lower him into his chair."

My prayers initially involved asking God for physical strength, decreased fatigue, the ability to lift Jay and his equipment, put on his braces, mow, and carry everything. Later, my prayers would involve the needs of emotional and spiritual strength. I also found myself asking God to help Jay recognize the difference between a medical touch and an intimate one, as I found myself struggling to balance my roles as caregiver and wife.

> I prayed for the strength to continue the work.
> —Nehemiah 6:9

These little prayers in the moments of need helped me realize how closely God attended to the details of our journey. He helped us every step of the way. I wonder how many angels in the Lord's army were there in our house with us to keep us going. Sometimes, God sent an angel of the human variety to our doorstep.

On September 9, 2005, Roland Cecil phoned to ask if he could visit. We were a bit restless at the time, still anxiously awaiting completion of our house construction. Jay's outlook brightened as soon as his visitor arrived. We had met Roland at church, where he greeted everyone prior to worship services and volunteered in the food pantry ministry. Roland sat near Jay's chair and read his handwritten poem, titled "Ode to Jay," which he had composed the day before.

In his own quiet, country gentleman's style, he told us God directs him to write poetry for special people in his life. There is only one copy, which now resides in my scrapbook, along with a photo of Roland as he read it to us. Roland has since passed away, but his kindness has left an indelible mark on my heart. His prose captured Jay's love for Christ and those around him. His gift came just when both of us needed a boost, and it motivated Jay to continue believing God still had a purpose for him to complete.

I might have known Jay's opportunities to speak publicly would continue to spring forth. Keeping up with both his spiritual exuberance and deteriorating condition was my constant challenge. He had become dependent on his wheelchair. But like one of those traveling country preachers of yesteryear, Jay was a circuit rider—on wheels!

Soon after Roland's visit, the ministerial staff of our megachurch contacted us about speaking in the worship series titled "Great Expectations," which they were planning for September and October of 2005. They commissioned Jay to share his journey "through the wilderness" with the church through a video.

Todd Carter, director of media ministry, came to our rental home to begin recording Jay's story on video. Todd interviewed both of us, along with Luke, for the vignette, which would be shown on the big screen as part of all the worship services! As of this writing, the pastoral staff of Ginghamsburg Church still use Jay's recorded testimony in presentations around the country. I continue to receive feedback about how it is globally ministering to people from all walks of life.

During the interview, Jay voiced his wonderment about how God was going to use this affliction in the future to impact others. He said:

> I hope that I'm (still) around to gain that "hindsight 20/20 vision" … to see what God does with this illness. I'd like to look back and say, "Ah! So that's what He had in mind!" I have great expectations, regardless of the outcome.

Jay and I were both so proud of Luke's courage and visionary, selfless thoughts about his father's terminal illness. In the "Great Expectations" segment, our son says, "Even if this disease claims my dad's life, he's going home. He gets the better end of the deal."

By mid-October, our house construction was finally complete, but Jay was already wheelchair-bound. Despite our trial-and-error construction experience, and a temporarily leaky fireplace gas line, we came through with beautiful results.

A few friends helped us prepare the finishing touches before we moved in. Larry Green hooked up Jay's computer and the TV. Luke and his friend hung towel bars in the bathroom to Jay's specifications. Under different circumstances, these were the things Jay might have done for someone else. Now others were coming to his aid.

During the third week of October, we unpacked our belongings and rejoiced over little things like not having to eat off plastic plates any longer. Friends celebrated with us and brought in food and helped us unpack. It was happy chaos! Laughter had entered our new home, as we unpacked (haphazardly), hung pictures, and shared meals over the first few days. We received cards from far and near, welcoming us to our new home.

Of course, the unspoken reality was that 2680 Stonebridge Drive was where Jay had come to die. But together with a few close friends from our cell group, we chose to celebrate life in this moment of victory. Pastor Mike Bowie led in blessing our home, and we shared Holy Communion in our living room. On that occasion, another video vignette was recorded for our church ministry.

When Jay was no longer able to sit at the dining table for meals, our friend Reid Sevitts created a special table that suited Jay's height, so he could eat with the family while remaining in his wheelchair. We purchased a wheelchair-accessible van. Reid played the guinea pig role, as we practiced using Jay's new Hoyer lift. I continued taking pictures of everyone who came into our home, and we always found something about which to laugh.

Our new home continued to be filled with visitors who rallied around Jay as though he were a rock star. We had game nights at the kitchen table, and Jay joined in. In November, our friends enabled us to attend the Casting Crowns Lifesong Concert Tour when it came to Dayton. We attended the 2005 ALS Walk Awards banquet and Christmas party, where Karen Wellbaum, family chair, presented the "Journey for Jay " team the second-place trophy for most money raised by an ALS team.

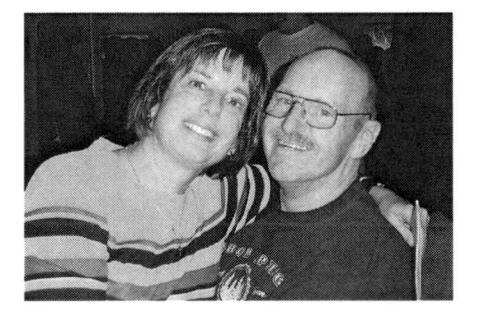

My favorite place to be; sitting on Jay's lap while he drove his chair

Now that Jay had become a public speaker and a poster child for Central and Southern Ohio's ALS Chapter, his "fame" seemed to know no bounds. We couldn't believe the number of people—strangers and friends alike—who offered to pray for us and help us in practical ways. Perhaps they didn't know *how* to help, but the concern was genuine and appreciated.

We had only just begun to understand that Jay's illness would take a community of caring people to help me help Jay to the finish line of his earthly life. I could not fathom how I would manage, as nerves in his body died and muscle degeneration continued. Jay's body became more sluggish and unresponsive with each passing day. But for now, we marveled at how strong Jay's testimony had become through adversity.

> I can do all things through Christ who strengthens me.
> —Philippians 4:13

CHAPTER SIX

HOSPICE ENTERS OUR VOCABULARY

Cruisin' for a Bruisin'

Publicly, Jay was a powerhouse of inspiration. Privately, he struggled to cope with his multiplying disabilities. Shortly after we moved into our house, he tried to flex his curled fingers for me to observe, but it was a pitiable effort. The broad, muscular hands that had served him well as a massage therapist had atrophied to something barely recognizable.

My heart broke—for Jay and for myself. Throughout our years together, my own hands had felt so small and safe in his. But with the awareness our time together was to be abbreviated, we never held hands as much as we did during Jay's illness. That comforting sense of human touch had become supremely important. We'd even hold each other's hand while drifting off to sleep each night.

As Jay lost use of his hands, I walked beside his wheelchair or sat in his lap and helped him drive by placing my hand over his to steer the chair. When he could no longer operate the controls at all, they were repositioned to the back, so I could be his requisite "backseat driver," so to speak.

Little did I know how challenging this would be! I had been warned it would be "different," but steering his chair from the back was like trying to do so in a house of mirrors. When I turned the controls right, the wheelchair went left, and vice versa. Maneuvering through tight spaces and entryways was impossible. I failed backseat driving miserably, because the chair would easily spin in circles, bump into the furniture and walls, and run over my toes. Jay and I were both at our wits' end.

> All those times that I thought I was in control in life and kept the Lord in the passenger seat, I get it now … I am never in control!"
> —Katie Jordan

As Thanksgiving approached, I knew instinctively we were entering a new phase of our journey with ALS. My strained back served as a constant reminder I was lifting more of his weight, as his own abilities were reduced and depleted. Despite all of our spiritually charged great expectations, Jay and I emotionally and physically struggled to endure.

I made an appointment with Dr. Laura Sams, who had coordinated Jay's medical care since the diagnosis. On Wednesday, November 30, 2005, after examining Jay, she solemnly recommended we contact hospice for Jay's care during his remaining time on Earth.

This jolting reality launched an adventurous, petulant holiday season of ups and downs. For one thing, when hospice first interviewed us, we were informed that Jay didn't qualify. As a caregiver, I challenged this determination, referencing Dr. Sams's recommendation. The hospice medical director informed us that to be further considered, we had to provide a list of the recent changes in his condition.

We included the following facts in our report to hospice administrators: (1) Jay could no longer operate our car under his handicapped license status; (2) he was confined to a wheelchair and could no longer rely on a walker; (3) atrophy had dramatically progressed in his dominant right hand and arm; (4) atrophy had appeared in his left hand and arm; (5) he now needed a bedrail; (6) Jay required moderate assistance when getting in and out of bed; (7) showering required assistance; (8) eating required assistance, and most important, (9) Jay was beginning to experience breathing problems in his sleep.

Miami County Hospice accepted us immediately after these clarifications. As a matter of fact, the hospice nurse predicted Jay would need a hospital bed within the month. With my persistence on Jay's behalf, we added a nurse and a social worker from hospice to our support team. The hospice chaplain phoned, offering his services as needed.

The primary caregiver is the patient's best advocate.
Persist!

The death process is much like the birth process. Jay was moving into Heaven's birth canal for his great exit. But there was still time for living. The process could not be escalated; nor could it be avoided. Only God knew the appointed hour or how we will cope in the meantime. Although we didn't know it, we had almost nineteen more months before Jay would draw his last breath.

A foreboding malaise swept over Jay as ALS continue to rob him of his dignity. I observed helplessly, as my usually upbeat Jay withdrew. When our friends were not around, Jay became despondent and uncommunicative, gazing out the window for hours.

He became irritable with me, as I placed the medications in his mouth, injected him, cut his meat for him, changed him, lifted him, and supervised orders for his care. Sometimes he snapped angrily, and I felt like an intruder with a big spotlight, revealing every indignity ALS had inflicted on him.

My own outlook was plunging into an abyss. I had ALS as much as Jay. Its indignities punished both of us. I no longer felt like Jay's wife, soul mate, and lover. Jay yelled at me for making all the decisions, and he proclaimed, "I'm damn tired of it."

A primary caregiver suffers as much at the hands
of terminal illness as her patient.
Grief is its name.

In years past, Jay had always known just what to say to encourage and uplift. He had always been my best cheerleader. But now we were lost in our grief and confusion, like children in a war zone. Our innocence had been obliterated. Everything we had been together before this disease entered our cognizance was gone. What had happened to our great expectations? Like a monster in the closet of our souls, grief came to reside in us. Jay was angry; I was scared.

Despite total exhaustion, I couldn't sleep at night. My mind couldn't turn off. I tossed in bed each night, mulling over a workable plan for the next day. I was caught in a vortex and spinning out of control. I needed to find a rejuvenation of spirit.

During the Christmas season of 2005, our most memorable gift was not found under the Christmas tree. My mother, who knew how much we had enjoyed traveling throughout our marriage, presented a gift of a seven-day Caribbean cruise.

To say the least, Jay and I had mixed emotions. Mom's gift was generous and thoughtful, meant to provide a respite from our confinement at home, to help us renew in the fresh sea air, see new sights, and experience one last trip together. Perhaps the change of scenery would be just what we needed.

As ridiculous as it seemed to imagine that this trip was doable, especially since Jay had just been approved by hospice, we accepted the challenge. Hospice agreed to postpone its services by one week, upon our return.

Jay and I both feared the unknowns, but he had been wishing we could take one last trip together, and here it was—our big chance. I prayed this cruise would ease my stress level and not increase it. I was about to navigate unknown waters: caregiving at sea. How's that for great expectations?

We decided Luke would have to come with us on our last getaway to help make transportation and life on a cruise ship possible. The flight connections would be quite challenging. We were scheduled for a cruise departing from Ft. Lauderdale, meaning we would fly from Dayton and change planes in Atlanta. We would visit the islands of Puerto Rico, St. Maarten, St. Thomas, Nassau, and port in Miami. From there, we would make the flight connections home again.

I spent a lot of time crying before we departed on December 11, 2005. With the addition of hospice care on the horizon, Jay's death sentence had become more real. As a caregiver, I was on an endless cycle of convincing myself I could handle the challenges, followed by a feeling of failure and exhaustion. Each time Jay's condition worsened, I'd have to start all over again, pumping up my strength and willpower to press on. What a time to go on a trip!

Photographs in my scrapbook bear proof that we somehow survived the cruise. Jay isn't smiling in most of the images, but we tried to do the touristy things. Luke and Jay played the slot machines, I had my hair braided in Nassau, and our Christmas card photo was taken as I posed on Jay's lap in his wheelchair in front of a giant outdoor Christmas tree in St. Maarten.

Jay and I stayed on the pier in St. Maarten, Nassau, and St. Thomas. We didn't even attempt to leave the ship in San Juan. During the week, we did some Christmas shopping and enjoyed the spa on board. Jay had two acupuncture treatments, which didn't help his condition, but he loved the attention. A facial temporarily gave me a healthy glow. I look at those pictures now and see how all three of us were trying to put on a happy face and just survive, but we felt completely out of place.

"A picture paints a thousand words," so the saying goes. One of the most telling photographs was of Jay, who had abandoned his wheelchair *by himself* and was pictured standing at the ship's railing, staring down into the murky waters, as if pondering whether to jump. I still can't believe we took this trip. Nor can I imagine how much pride Jay had to swallow, as we had stepped way out on a limb to take one last vacation.

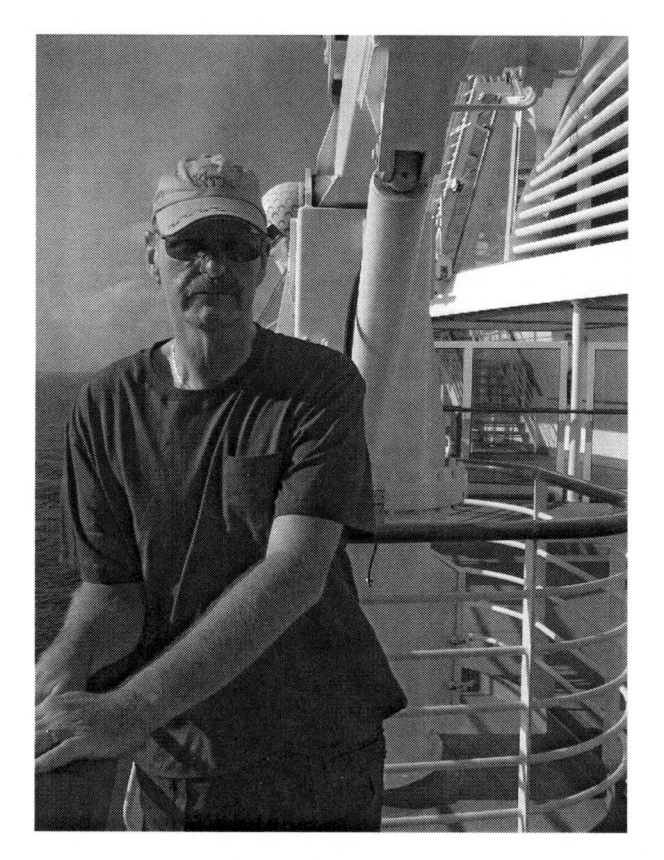

The picture says it all

Although the cruise line claimed to have handicapped accessibility, it was very basic at best. Our bathroom had bars, but the bed was extremely low, making it very difficult to manage Jay's care. Also, maneuvering Jay through our quarters in his wheelchair was impossible due to all the furniture packed into the tiny space. When I asked the steward to remove the excess furnishings, he refused, citing the cruise line's policy.

Guest Relations on board had a pat answer for everything we requested: "Sorry."

"Sorry, there are no excursions tailored for the disabled."

"Sorry, the elevators are broken."

"Sorry about the furniture problem in your room."

Luke and I put our creative minds together and produced a temporary solution to the cramped living quarters. Never mind that a couple of pieces of excess furniture got a sea spray bath on our room's balcony. We returned everything to its proper place upon our departure.

However, angels were on board with us in the form of our waiter, Glen, and a guest who was an occupational therapist, who offered to help us lift Jay off a lounge chair; I couldn't manage on my own. What would we have done without the help of passengers who volunteered to help us maneuver Jay's wheelchair up and down the ramps?

Jay remarked this was the first time he had ever felt discriminated against. Disheartened, he declared he had traveled for the last time.

> Save me, O God, for the waters have come up to my neck.
> I sink in the miry depths, where there is no foothold.
> I have come into the deep waters; the floods engulf me.
> I am worn out calling for help; my throat is parched.
> My eyes fail, looking for my God.
> —Psalm 69:1–3

As soon as we returned home, we met with the intake nurse from hospice. She was visibly shocked at the changes in Jay's condition. His transfer skills in and out of bed were nonexistent. He needed help dressing and began using a bath chair for the shower. Jay blamed the phlegm in the back of his throat for changes in his voice, but at this point, his lungs were still clear. An aide was assigned to come to our home to bathe and dress him Monday through Friday, which was a real blessing.

The hospice chaplain and a hospice LPN came to visit us. At one point, they took me aside in the garage for a private consultation about Jay's health. In addition, I received lots of hugs, encouragement, and their shoulders to cry on. I'm sure they did this type of ministry all the time, but I certainly didn't feel like "another number" at all and am very grateful for their compassionate assistance.

With the cruise now in the past, our next challenge was to survive the holidays. People were pouring in and out of our home as if it were Grand Central Station. Jay's family visited from Kentucky, our children came, and my parents and sister popped in. On top of that, we had the usual plethora of Jay's supporters, friends, and aides, which now included hospice staff. I wonder if we should have installed a revolving door during the house construction? Of course, we were grateful for every visit and celebrated Christ's birthday and laughed in spite of the circumstances. But inside, I felt lost at sea with no safe port in which to dock.

Although I had decorated the new house for the holidays, it still felt sterile, like a hospital. I had looked forward to my children's involvement in placing finishing touches on the Christmas tree and embellishing the new house with our cache of family memories and pictures. Sarah flew in from California, and Matt came from New York. Luke, who attended an area college, had followed his dad's condition more closely since before the diagnosis.

For Sarah and Matt, I had imagined and hoped for cheerful visits with Jay. Instead, a cold feeling of dreaded anticipation gripped me, as I realized by Sarah's and Matt's body language the depth of their pain. They clearly were not totally able to conceive of or reconcile the seriousness of Jay's condition. They certainly didn't talk to me about their feelings, and I didn't talk to them about mine. If we had addressed these topics, we might have cried through Christmas.

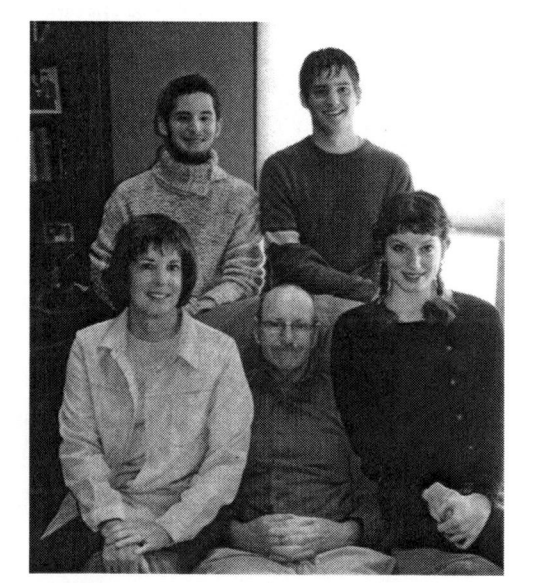

Our family picture taken Christmas 2005

Jay was a wonderful father and stepfather and voiced his pride in Sarah, Matthew Asher (whom he affectionately called Masher), and Luke. Following the holidays, he seemed to evaluate each of the children's reactions. He said, "I kind of wonder how my kids are doing psychologically. I don't want anyone feeling guilty or thinking they didn't do enough when I was alive. I don't need anyone going down that road. It doesn't accomplish a darn thing."

On my birthday, December 30, I took Jay out to celebrate over dinner before we went to church. He couldn't lift his glass. The expression on Jay's face was so sad. He lamented that he couldn't even buy me a card. I wanted to cheer him up, but I felt as helpless as he did. It was as though we were in some foreign place, where everything seemed wrong. The spirit to make these efforts was going out of us.

As I always did when that sinking feeling loomed, I wrote prayers in my journal, confessing to the Lord that I clearly couldn't take care of Jay in my own strength. Deciding on my New Year's resolution was easy: to give the controls of my life back to God. It was the only way I could ride the currents of 2006 ... and the only way to be present for Jay.

NEW YEAR'S PRAYER

Dear God,
Bless all our friends with good things this coming year.
If we can't get out into the community,
let us continue to touch others in any way You see fit.
May we be an inspiration to those around us.
Most of all, bring the right people into my kids' lives
so that they can feel your light and love through them.
I ask for this peaceful feeling to continue to
come over me when I need it the most.
Please allow me to see the Angels that are all around us.
Amen.

CHAPTER SEVEN

THE SERMON THAT CHANGED EVERYTHING

We Carried the Mat Is Born

By January of 2006, Jay's increasing muscle spasticity had given way to immobility. We relied on a growing arsenal of home health equipment to assist us in preparing him for an outing.

After our cruise, Jay never used his walker again. While I could still help him to a standing position to shift from his bed to his chair, he was either not interested or unable to take steps. I finally decided to confront him about walking. He said he didn't feel safe with just me to assist him, so at the support group meeting, I asked Pinky to help "spot" him, and we observed as he made attempts to use the walker. He legs scissored, and finally, he sat down and said, "This is not going to work."

I gave the walker back to the ALS Association's loan closet, so it could be loaned out to someone else. Getting him in and out of bed was an ordeal. His fatigue and stiffness increased with each passing day. Therapeutic assistance I could administer as a physical therapist were no longer effective.

From the time my feet hit the floor in the morning until I closed my eyes at night, sometimes too exhausted to sleep, my days were a jumble of nursing tasks. I would drop one chore to pick up two others and lose myself in the shuffle.

Even leaving Jay long enough to take a shower became risky. I'd make Jay promise he would stay in bed until I was finished bathing. Even when he earnestly promised, I couldn't trust him. More often than not, I would find him trying to sit up on the side of the bed before I could get dressed. So, I would stop dressing to go and help him into his chair.

Each day was fitful with anticipation of a fall waiting to happen. Lifting Jay became increasingly difficult and scary. I was terrified he would slip from my grip and onto the floor. Eventually, I began to use a transfer belt when lifting and transferring him. Finally, he forbade me from trying to lift him by myself. Some evenings, if no one was present to assist with bedtime preparations, that meant he had to sleep in his chair in the living room.

Although I tried to put on a brave face for Jay and our loved ones, my soul was becoming consumed with fear. I was afraid for Jay, but I was equally afraid for myself. We could no longer share our innermost thoughts. Jay didn't yet feel comfortable discussing last wishes and funeral arrangements with me. I secretly worried about what I would do when that time came. I wondered if the community support would still be there for me after Jay's death. After all, he was the popular one who drew crowds. What was going to happen to me?

Throughout our married life, I had been able to confide completely my heart's concerns to Jay. Until now. We had always been able to talk about any situation. ALS had stripped this element of intimacy from our experience. Now, in the face of Jay's terminal illness, my own welfare and concerns were promptly placed on the back burner in order for me to be truly present for him. This unresolved stress swelled within, interrupting sleep, as I tried to cope with the multiple rudimentary tasks of Jay's care. I was on a roller coaster that had no end in sight.

Well-meaning friends and acquaintances who came and went sometimes offered to lend a listening ear, but I remember sensing they couldn't help unless they had walked in my shoes, so why burden them? Who would have understood? People were always advising me, "Take a hot bath," or some such solution. I was worried how I could find the time to eat and go to the bathroom, much less take a hot bath. The bottom line was that no one truly understood we were under siege, and death was the enemy.

Jay and I didn't have much more time together. Our lives had been consumed with ALS at its ugliest. Our house seemed to have become a hospital, with people coming in and out without end. We had no privacy, yet we were totally isolated. I sometimes wanted to reach out to someone for help, but it was exhausting to speak to someone for assistance.

> *Caregivers need help in providing care for their loved one,*
> *so they can also take care of themselves.*
> *Most people would like to assist but need guidance.*
> *Share your needs and those of your loved one,*
> *so they can be part of the solution.*

A laborious, multistep process had to take place before we could go for a drive, take Jay for a therapeutic swim at the YMCA, attend a medical appointment, have dinner with friends, or attend a worship service. Jay had to be taken to the bathroom, exercised, bathed, dressed, fed, and transported. Over time, we had developed quite a routine that sapped both hours from our day and all the strength I could muster. My muscles ached, and my back felt as though it would break each time I placed him into the Hoyer lift and transported him to bed, bathroom, wheelchair, or easy chair. So, in transporting Jay to church and other outings, we gladly accepted Luke's offers to assist us with transfers and driving and parking our van.

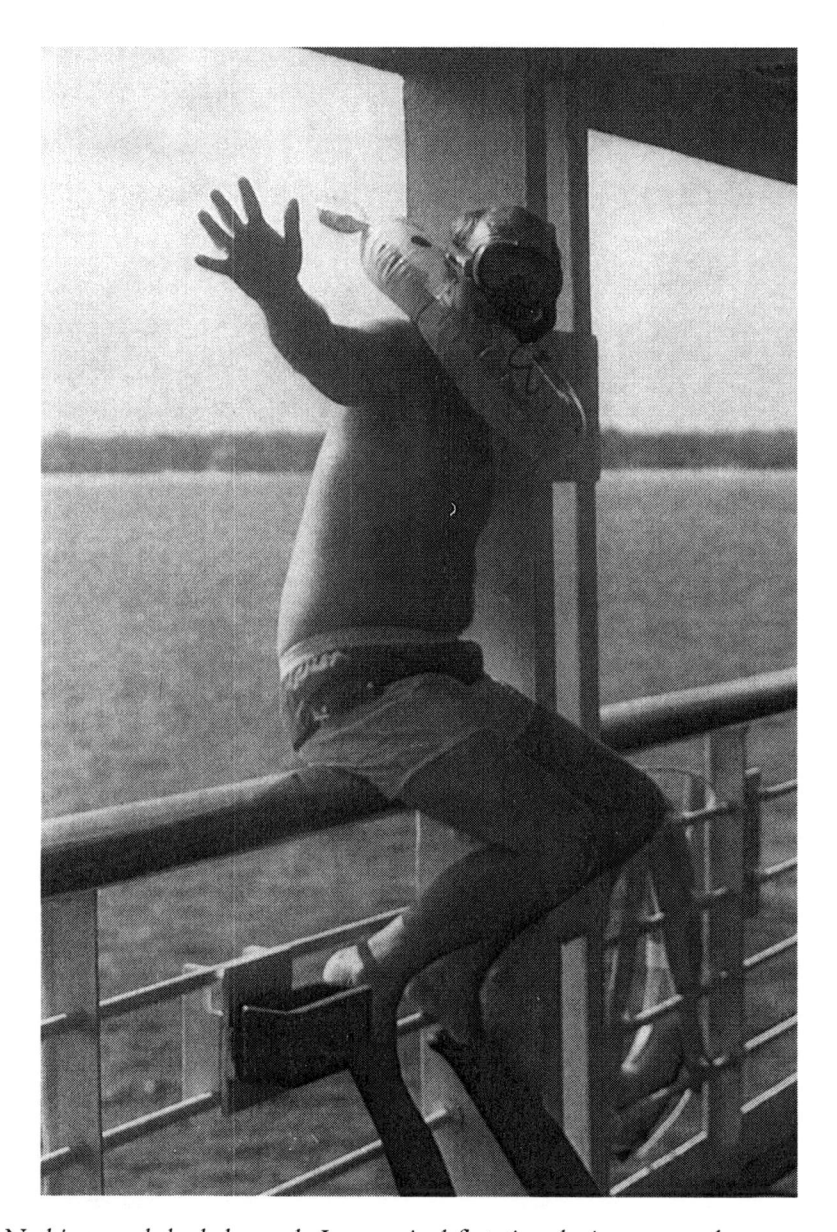

Nothing much had changed; Jay required flotation devices on our honeymoon

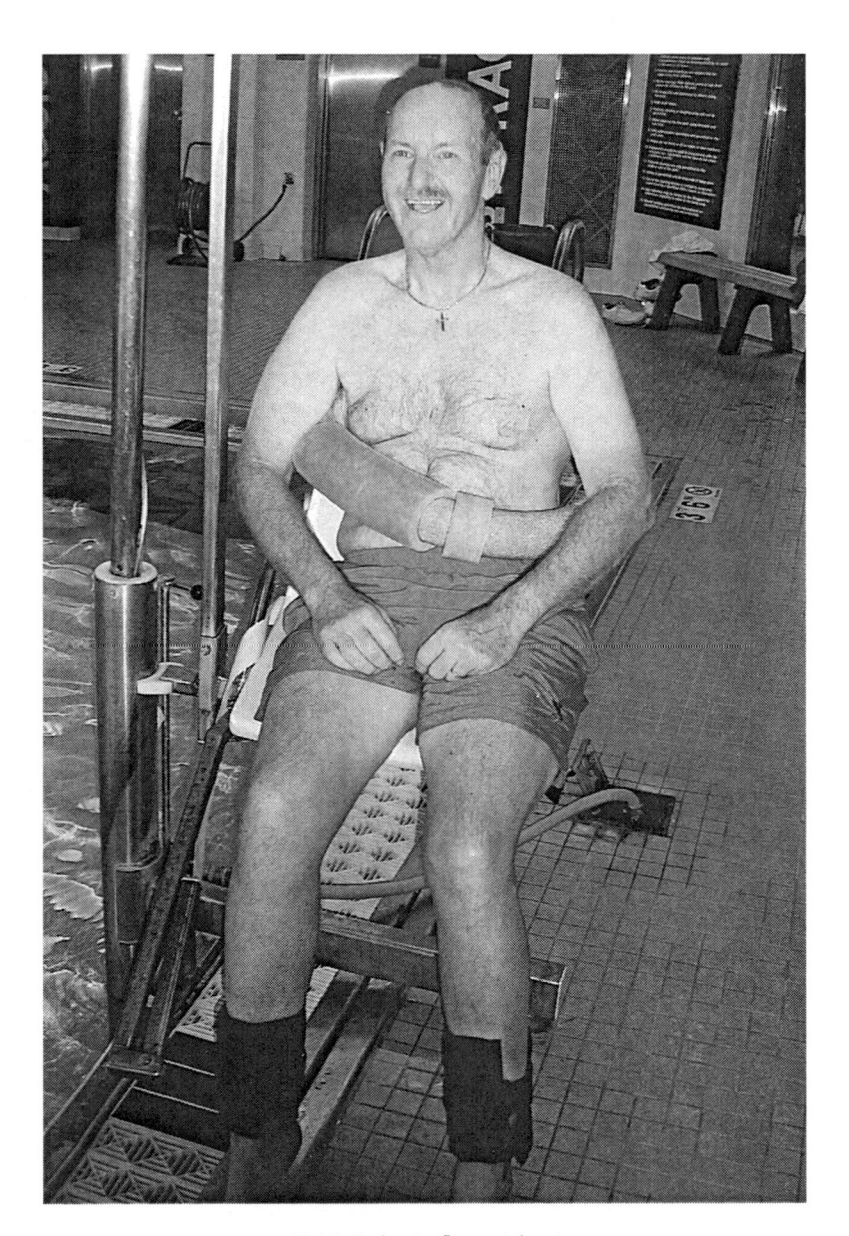

PALS don't float either!

Anywhere we went, by the time we arrived, I'd be ready for a nap. Meanwhile, Jay would be all smiles for his adoring public. I would manage to "paste" on a tired, plastic smile, while people beelined to greet Jay. He heartily received their hugs and best regards.

For years, Jay's genuine faith and clever turn of a phrase had endeared him to many people through his professional and personal connections alike. As a kind and personable Bible teacher, he had brought life to the stories of Jesus and His followers. Over the years, many people had sought him out for his gifted ability to apply the scriptures to daily life with anecdotes and a touch of humor. People, including me, craved his natural charisma. They would tell him what an inspiration he was and that they were so glad he came.

Meanwhile, as Jay held court with his admirers like a decadent king, I felt banned to the tower of isolation. Whether our acquaintances and friends were aware they avoided eye contact with me, I will never know. But Jay was clearly their interest.

Of course, it pleased me that Jay was welcomed anywhere we went with smiles of encouragement and accolades of kindness. I tried to tell myself it was only natural. He was the one with the terminal illness, and he wouldn't be with us much longer. Perhaps they felt compelled to direct their attentions toward him while they could. Yet, despite my feeble attempts at positive self-talk, I couldn't deny feeling neglected. I was also hurt that Jay privately exhibited impatience with me, as we struggled through our strenuous daily routine. My silent pain began to hurt more and more. Luke and I always found ourselves in the same place over and over again: in the shadows of Jay's entourage of support. How I ached for affirmation and compassion as Jay's primary caregiver and wife. No one seemed to know the cost to me to get him there and that the two-hour process would be repeated once we left for home. Aside from that, didn't they know I felt terrified and alone?

Caregivers are vulnerable to depression and isolation.
Emotional support through prayer, encouragement, and friendship can help.
Make your needs known.

As Jay was swamped with admirers, the truth washed over me: we were no longer a "couple" to our friends. The curse of a terminal prognosis was even redefining our friendships with others. What more would ALS do to sever our lives into little pieces? Did I have to lose my identity in the community, too?

Fear enveloped me, as I realized the challenges ahead would only intensify. Early on, I could literally see Jay dying a little bit every day. He would lose some movement or develop a new symptom. When his condition bottomed out, how would I manage? How I longed for comfort from our friends.

On a particular Saturday evening, January 20, 2006, I positioned Jay's wheelchair at the front of the church and sank into the pew for worship ... to hear the sermon that would change everything. Our friend and senior pastor, Mike Slaughter, began his message, which struck me at the very heart of my need for affirmation and physical help in managing Jay's care.

Mike stressed the importance of community, as described in Mark 2:1–8, in which four supportive friends of a paralyzed man transported their friend, lying on a simple makeshift bed or mat, to the place where Jesus of Nazareth was preaching. They knew if they could just transport their friend to Jesus, He would heal him.

The familiar story was a balm to my aching spirit, as Mike continued. When the friends carrying the mat couldn't access the building due to the crowds of people who packed in to hear Jesus, they didn't give up. They managed to climb to the roof with their afflicted friend in tow. They dug a hole in the roof and lowered the mat to the feet of God's Son. Jesus stopped speaking. He looked at the paralyzed man lying on the mat and then up at the friends, who peered hopefully through the hole in the roof.

Upon seeing the great faith of the paralyzed man's friends, Jesus healed him.

By the time Mike reached this point in his sermon, Jay, Luke, and I were sobbing. We could see ourselves in that scripture passage! Jay was on the mat, and Luke and I were carrying him to Jesus. But we needed help.

Our minister wasn't finished. He noted the scripture states the man's healing occurred supernaturally because of the faith of his friends. The paralyzed man's *community* of support had persevered in helping the man get to Jesus. By *their* faith, he was healed.

Pastor Mike then looked at Jay and smiled. We smiled back through our tears. We had been the illustration of today's sermon! We were meeting Jesus through Mike's message. *Perhaps now,* I thought, *the church family will come alongside me and help carry Jay's mat.* For the first time in a long time, I felt hopeful. This sermon was a lifeline for Jay, our son, and me in our need!

I wasn't a bit surprised when Mike invited Jay to come forward, so the "community of believers" could come forward to pray for his healing. But I was very surprised and hurt he didn't ask Luke and me to come forward for prayer as well. People rushed to pray over Jay in a great outpouring of love. Meanwhile, Luke and I had been overlooked again. Again we were in the shadows. As I sat in the church pew, I wept for all the caregivers of spouses, parents, or children who are carrying the mat for their loved one but who are being neglected in their human experience and pain. A family friend near me whispered, "You need to talk to the pastor. Tell him how you feel."

I went home that day, hurt and angry, pondering how to deal with my turmoil in a positive way. Pastor Mike was an admired family friend and a spiritual leader with global influence. A few days later, I wrote him a message. I began by thanking him for the poignant illustration in his sermon and for the church's prayers for Jay.

Then I lowered the boom and boldly suggested he had missed the point of his own message! Like the afflicted man's faithful friends, I wrote, Luke and I were Jay's caregivers, also in need of acknowledgment and affirmation. As Jay's reliance on me increased, I had reached a crisis point. Carrying Jay's mat alone was becoming impossible. I needed prayer and practical help to carry Jay's mat to Heaven's gate.

> O Lord, you have examined my heart and
> know everything about me.
> You know when I sit down or stand up,
> You know my every thought when far away.
> You chart the path ahead of me and tell me where to stop and rest.
> Every moment you know where I am.
>
> —Psalm 139:1–3

To be honest, I didn't think my message would be taken seriously. But I felt better having shared my feelings with Mike. Although he didn't respond directly, things started to happen.

First, John Jung, Jay's mentor on the church staff, phoned and asked for the first time, "How are you, Katie?" He began visiting us frequently, taking an interest in the entire family.

Pastor Mike Slaughter's wife, Carolyn, called me as well. She asked what the church could do to help me provide care for Jay. I expressed that my most difficult time was at night, trying to get Jay ready for bed.

As a result, Carolyn placed a plea in the church bulletin. Several volunteers with nursing degrees and other skilled medical training responded. Before I knew it, church member Janie Rowlett, a registered nurse, coordinated a rotating schedule for the nurses to help me get Jay in bed each night.

By March 2006, we had a small army of bedtime assistants, who Jay dubbed the Night Angels. They would serve faithfully for the last fifteen months of Jay's life. Their tasks began around 9 p.m. and lasted an hour to an hour and a half. They brushed his teeth, washed his face, changed his clothes, administered his medications, flushed his tubes, and transferred him to bed.

But something else miraculous happened between our Night Angels and us. They became members of our extended family. Aside from the usual routine, they delighted Jay by coming early and giving me a break. They would pet and bring treats for our dog, Tipper, sing, dance, share a few jokes, and feed Jay Popsicles. They spent long hours talking with him, praying with him, bringing in food to share, and sleeping over.

Before it was over, some of our Night Angels recruited their husbands, who would eventually become so close to Jay they were named his pallbearers. Being ever the humorist of the bunch, Jay nicknamed his Night Angels as follows:

Jay's Night Angels

Janie "HMFIC" Rowlette, Chief Angel
Scott "Suction Scott" Rowlette, Chief Angel
Tori "Hillbilly" Peck
Ruth "Here Comes the Boogie Man" Gaines
Deb "The Quiet One" Meyer
Jim "The Dog Whisperer" Meyer
Beth "The Tooth Fairy" or "Dancing Queen" Thoele
Kathy "Magellan" Conrad
Reed Sevitts (nickname confidential to protect the innocent!)
Donna "Turkey Baster Queen" Sevitts
Lynne "Doo-Dad" Cox
Chuck "Biscuit" or "I Shot The Sheriff" Cox

Some wouldn't want their Jay-dubbed names listed here. They are just a little too personal, but you get the idea. There seemed to be no secrets among this special breed of caregivers. Jay's advancing symptoms were scary, but Jay led the charge in dispensing our fears by affirming his angels with funny names and quips only we could fully appreciate. They became our extended family, and through the laughter and banter, sometimes Jay would let down his guard and share his heart.

Do not forget to entertain strangers, for by doing so,
some people have entertained angels without knowing it.
—Hebrews 13:2

Another beautiful gift the Night Angels gave me was affirmation. In truth, I cannot remember how many offers they made to let me take a break and get out of the house. In the beginning, I could not bring myself to accept them. I assume that's why God kept sending people to reason with me. Besides, I'm sure I must have looked like I needed a break! In truth, my back and hips were aching from the abuse they were taking from Jay's daily care. I also felt trapped inside four walls. I would have angry days, when death and dying were all we ate, breathed, and talked about. It was conquering both of us, not just Jay, and I felt unable to do anything about it.

With these kinds of thoughts swirling about and the workload of Jay's care increasing, I was losing sight of a healthy mind-set. I thought perhaps those men in the little white coats were going to come and whisk me away in a straitjacket if something didn't change soon! Then I remembered something Pastor Sue Kibbey had said when we confided with her about Jay's condition:

In this season of your life, you need to allow others to serve you. That is of value to God.

I resolved thereafter to accept their offers to get out of the house or to lie down for a few minutes, even if napping was impossible. Of all people, Jay knew how stressed and tired I was. I could trust certain friends and the Night Angels with his care and knew this was God's gift to me. Besides, the act of "refilling my cup" meant I had something positive to give Jay when I returned to him.

> *Caregivers need personal time to rejuvenate.*
> *Taking time away is not selfish.*
> *Continue to take time for an activity you enjoy.*
> *Have a wish list ready when someone asks what he or she can do to help.*

The outings were great, once I began accepting the opportunities offered. However, I inherited another problem: high separation anxiety. As I drove home each time, a little wave of panic would wash over me.

I wondered what I would find. Dirty dishes? Jay on the floor? Extra people to feed? A messy house to clean up?

I learned from comparing notes with other caregivers that this concern is normal. One day, when we were heading to our cars following worship, Bobette's husband, Jeff, and Patti Green, whose husband was also ill, expressed similar concerns. We concluded, right there in the parking lot, that getting out was worth the risk and that typically, we found our spouses to be comfortable on our return.

As I became comfortable with the idea of taking time for myself, I wearied of having to repeat instructions over and over again to the kind caregivers who flooded into our home. So, I began writing notes with morning care instructions for those who volunteered to bathe, dress, and perform dental hygiene routines. As Jay's needs became more complicated, I developed a laminated bullet list for the morning. When the Night Angels were added, I added a similar list of evening care instructions for them to follow. These were posted in the bathroom, bedroom, and kitchen.

Lists began to grow like weeds in a garden, as I wrote out patient care instructions for bowel and bladder, the feeding tube, multiple uses of the hospital bed, the Hoyer lift, and later, the Bi-PAP. In the fullness of time, the laminator became my new best friend.

I had peace of mind if I was away from Jay for an hour or two, knowing these instructions were readily available to whoever was "on call." In addition, the doors were never locked at our house, so in the event of an emergency, we could have more-immediate assistance.

> As Jay's condition progressed and our need for quiet grew,
> signs were occasionally added on the door, such as:
> "We are recharging our batteries ... please, no visitors today."

On one of my first outings, Jay happily entertained a couple of visitors. My destination? The church's New Path. It was such an emotional release to be able to share my heart with three compassionate staff members who listened, truly cared, and prayed with me.

While there, I ran into Bill Duff, the director of New Path, who gave me such a lift when he looked into my eyes and said, "Katie, you and your [children] need prayers just as much as Jay does."

What a gift for my soul! It was the first time anyone had voiced that truth to me. My heart had hungered for such affirmation, and here it was! I can't express how much lighter I felt when I returned home to Jay with that sense of self-worth tucked into my heart. Such compassion and validation in Bill's kind statement had energized me. I felt valued! To this day, that experience fuels my passion for ministry to the needs of weary caregivers.

Caregivers perform immeasurable amounts of difficult, important work and need validation, understanding, and reassurance.

While Jay could still communicate but was becoming more dependent on me, our every need was met through a community of mat carriers. Through the story in Pastor Mike's sermon and what transpired thereafter, I realized I had a story to tell. Not a happily-ever-after kind of story, but the story of the trials and joys of the primary caregiver and those who came alongside her in the toughest assignment anyone can be given.

And to think—it all started with a sermon.

CHAPTER EIGHT

FACING OUR FEARS/ COPING WITH ANGER

It Must Have Been the Frogs ...

During the winter of 2006, Jay alternated between his wheelchair and lift chair. Hospice aides, our Night Angels, and others from the medical community routinely came and went from our home to assist me with his round-the-clock care. Jay and I had become victims engaged in siege warfare with ALS. We were grateful to have these mat carriers in the trench with us, because the fight was more rigorous than my body could have withstood.

The droning routines of lifting, bathing, and fretting over frequent infections, nighttime breathing problems, and choking spells continued for the rest of his life. My days and nights were threaded together with rudimentary duties that allowed no time for rest.

We both sensed the crescendo of death's sluggish but certain approach. Underlying swells of concern and high anxiety threatened to surface, though I strived to keep my personal grief from showing. I felt Jay needed a caregiver and wife with a cheerful disposition, no matter what. Yet, there was no denying the heartache. His affliction had now incapacitated every area of our lives. Even our most intimate moments were coming to an end. His last attempts to make love to me had been bewildering, sad, and bittersweet.

After he could no longer hold and caress me, I would sometimes purposefully envelop myself in his arms and close my eyes. We would lie together, wrapped in a precious few moments of wistful, sentimental, heartbreaking silence. These attempts at intimacy reminded Jay I was still his wife, not just his nursemaid and caregiver. I too needed his touch to remind me he was my beloved husband, although he lay trapped in a listless, unresponsive body. I tried to conceal my weeping for the way our life together used to be.

Neither of us knew how to broach difficult issues related to his death and dying, or how to meet each other's needs for reassurance and comfort. Perhaps it was just too much of an effort to exhume our worst fears, so we most often chose to keep them buried. However, one night, not long after Jay's birthday in late February 2006, I climbed into Jay's hospital bed, where we watched the Olympics together. Snuggling close with the TV on helped us recapture a bit of normality. It became a rare opportunity for us to engage in a heart-to-heart talk, during which my growing fears unfurled like a tidal wave.

Jay listened intently. I explained that until recently, I had felt well equipped to provide his required level of care by virtue of my physical therapy training. But now that his illness had progressed to a more-advanced stage, I felt afraid. He had recently choked twice, as he attempted to chew and swallow food. His nighttime respiration was compromised, meaning at times, he wasn't getting enough oxygen. As a result of being honest with him and confronting my fears, Jay consented to having a percutaneous endoscopic gastrostomy (PEG) tube, or feeding tube, surgically inserted directly into his abdomen for nourishment.

As it turned out, my admission of fear seemed to open the door for Jay to open his heart to me. He brought up the need to plan his funeral. He confessed he'd been afraid I would think he was giving up if he talked about finalizing his funeral. I confessed my relief at his decision, because pre-planning would grant our minds some measure of peace. We cried together and felt closer than we had in a long time.

From performing the most menial task, to asking hospice for a hospital bed, to having procedures like the surgical insertion of a PEG tube, each challenge was a hurdle we crossed into the unknown. Jay and I aspired to meet every fear we had with brute faith: the faith we had learned and talked about in our Bible studies with friends or in our daily devotions from years past. Now, we were putting these lessons to the test in a battle of life and death. God was faithfully showing us how to prepare for the end ... one step at a time.

I cried out to the Lord, and He answered me,
freeing me from all my fears.
—Psalm 34:4

It Must Have Been the Frogs

When life as we had known it was under attack, we proposed to live each day with consistent faith and trust in God, no matter what. How timely that a friend sent us a card in the spring of 2006 about the importance of, "putting on the full armor of God," to protect us from all harm.

At the time, Jay was taking seventy-two pills per day. His physical complications continued to progress. His personality underwent subtle changes. He didn't seem to realize how much he rambled, more than likely due to his decreased oxygen.

On occasion, he would lash out and say hurtful things to the aide on duty, as well as to me. We knew these verbal reactions were not really directed at us. Jay even confessed privately that he might have some brain involvement with the ALS progression.

He began sleeping more and became unable to drive his wheelchair. As I described in a previous chapter, it was quite an adventure to steer the chair from behind. We hit walls and ran over toes, and in the process, our tempers grew shorter fuses.

Bowel, bladder, swallowing, and respiration functions had become increasingly impaired. Meanwhile, Jay spoke more openly of death, and he admitted his fear of leaving me alone. I tried to tell him I'd be fine but would always cry. Emotions were swirling frantically for both of us. My back pain was at a maximum from so much lifting. Jay's abilities had decreased to an all-time low, and I felt that I was running on empty.

On April 21, 2006, Jay met with our pulmonologist, Dr. Younger, and failed two tests. Dr. Younger called hospice, and by Wednesday, we had a Bi-PAP machine and a quick lesson on how to use it.

In addition to hospice staff present daily, we were still completing details on our home. Landscape fencers worked in the backyard, along with concrete layers who were putting in patios and sidewalks. A sprinkler system was being installed. And we lost two of our best Night Angels: Ruth Gaines (who has since died) and Kathy Conrad. At that time, two new aides came from Upper Valley Medical Center to help with Jay's care.

Meanwhile, our friend Bobette was losing her battle with cancer, as it spread throughout her body. I longed to spend time with her. Another friend, Catherine Gohrband, had pneumonia for six weeks, and I wished I could be of help to her.

What a time for me to be completing my lifecare planning certification! However, with Jay's condition worsening by the minute, we both felt it was important that I anticipate how I could financially and professionally survive on my own. Final tests were approaching in June, so I also had to find time each day to study.

I forgot all about putting on the full armor of God, as the scripture in the card had advised. Everything on all fronts had come to a head. In short, I was ready to explode from all the pressure. So I did.

The trigger?
Sometimes it is the tiniest thing—even a little frog.
Thousands of them.

The neighborhood development where we were building our house had developed a drainage problem —and with it, an influx of tiny frogs. Adjacent to our lot was a swampy habitat for a legion of happy little polliwogs. Now that they sported brand new legs, they were leaving the comforts of their watery home to invade ours.

Their migration seemed to happen overnight. The amphibious trespassers sunbathed on our brand-new sidewalks and invaded the flowerbeds our friends had put in for us. They were suctioned onto our picture windows, napping on doorsills, and a squadron even found a way to invade the garage.

It was a plague of frogs no less dramatic than the one faced by the Egyptians in Biblical days, when Pharaoh refused to allow Moses and his people to return to Israel.

> Then the Lord said to Moses,
> "Go to Pharaoh once again and tell him,
> 'This is what the LORD says: Let my people go,
> so they can worship me.
> If you refuse, then listen carefully to this;
> I will send vast hordes of frogs across your entire land
> From one border to the other.
> The Nile River will swarm with them.
> They will come up out of the river and into your houses,
> Even into your bedrooms and onto your beds!
> Every home in Egypt will be filled with them.
> They will fill even your ovens and your kneading bowls.
> You and your people will be overwhelmed by frogs!"
> Then the LORD said to Moses,
> "Tell Aaron to point his shepherd's staff toward all the rivers,
> canals, and marshes of Egypt
> So there will be frogs in every corner of the land."
> Aaron did so, and frogs covered the whole land of Egypt!
> —Exodus 8:1–6

We were overwhelmed with frogs, just like the Egyptians experienced when old, hard-hearted Pharaoh wouldn't let Moses and God's people go. I think ALS is a lot like a plague of frogs. Those thousands of little frogs had pushed my last button—broken the last straw—plucked my last string. My rage erupted, and I pitched the most volcanic hissy fit imaginable. It was either the frogs or me!

Meanwhile, Jay, now a quadriplegic, watched helplessly from underneath a blanket in his easy chair near the picture window, where a number of little green creatures from the lagoon had attached themselves. I ranted and raved at the top of my lungs, as I swatted the unwelcome guests with brooms and towels. I startled them by swinging the door open. I slammed the doors closed to make them hop away. But I didn't stop there.

I told Jay I was moving out. I didn't care where. I had worked day and night. I had been a slave to ALS, and I was finished. I just wanted out.

Actually, in the end, I stayed, because lashing at those silly frogs turned out to be therapeutic. Tiny frog carnage remained plastered to the sidewalk, until a few summer rains washed the evidence of my mass murder away.

The Bible says God sent the plague of frogs to "encourage" Pharaoh to let the Israelites go out of slavery and into the Promised Land. Our frogs might have hopped out of that drainage pool as God's reminder He was there to help "encourage," even rescue, me (us) from our slavery to disease.

"Let my people go!"

God gave me such a release of emotion during that crisis. Since then, the wet yard issues were resolved. As we spent time in our yard, I began to spot ladybugs. I remembered a time shortly after Jay's diagnosis, when I'd asked God to show me a sign—ladybugs—to prove He cared

and knew what we faced. I was reminded the Lord's abiding grace was
ever-present.

Be strong with the Lord's mighty power.
Put on all of God's armor so that you will be able to stand firm
against all strategies and tricks of the Devil.
For we are not fighting against people made of flesh and blood,
but against the evil rulers and authorities of the unseen world,
against those mighty powers of darkness who rule this world,
and against wicked spirits n the heavenly realms.
Use every piece of God's armor to resist
the enemy in the time of evil,
so that after the battle you will still be standing firm.
Stand your ground, putting on the sturdy belt of truth
and the body armor of God's righteousness.
For shoes, put on the peace that comes from the Good News,
so that you will be fully prepared.
In every battle you will need faith as your shield
to stop the fiery arrows aimed at you by Satan.
Put on salvation as your helmet,
and take the sword of the Spirit, which is the word of God.
Pray at all times and on every occasion in
the power of the Holy Spirit.

—Ephesians 6:10–18

CHAPTER NINE

UNEXPECTED JOYS

The Flamingo Escapade
Trophy Wife Status
US Air Lands in Our Home
Jailhouse Rock

After the plague of frogs fiasco, I was determined to lighten up. An evening of fun with friends, designed to help us forget our troubles, was long overdue!

On a balmy summer's night, an undercover party operation was launched that I'll refer to as "the Flamingo Escapade." My motive was to create an evening in which the participants, two of whom were terminally ill, didn't have to think about death and dying. For a while, we could be carefree and not worry about financial and medical burdens. The laughter and camaraderie would rejuvenate us.

Our friends Bob and Marilyn Freeman were out of town on a Caribbean vacation. Jay and I, along with Reed and Donna Sevitts, and Jeff and Bobette Borchardt, decided that since the Freemans hadn't invited us to go along with them, we would make use of their grounds while they were away.

Our mini-vacation destination was the water fountain in their front yard followed by a photo session at their hot tub on the back porch.

Sporting swimwear and Mexican hats while sipping tropical beverages, we swore the house-sitters to secrecy about our little fiesta. We planted pink flamingoes on the premises as our calling card and left a wheelchair trail in our wake. Only a CSI investigator (Bob) was capable of solving our happy little crime once he and Marilyn arrived home from their vacation. They were greatly amused and most gracious. Mission accomplished! Fun was had by all, and the proof is in the pictures.

> There is a time for everything,
> a season for every activity under heaven.
> A time to be born and a time to die.
> A time to plant and a time to harvest.
> A time to kill and a time to heal.
> A time to tear down and a time to rebuild.
> A time to cry and a time to laugh.
> A time to grieve and a time to dance.
> —Ecclesiastes 3:1–4

We enjoyed surprise visits from Jay's former US Air colleagues who were in Dayton, Ohio, for a reunion. Many of them decided to stop in and pay us a visit. Later, Jay told everyone who came to our house that US Air had landed in our home.

Among those coming to talk old times with Jay were: Ed and Liz Johnson of Orlando, Florida; Jay's former boss, Wayne Rankin of Ashville, North Carolina; Bonnie and Jim Watkins of Myrtle Beach, South Carolina; David "Hummer" Johnson of Natural Bridge, Kentucky; and "Fast Eddie" Johnson, Julie Whittington, Larry Green, and Mark Wilson. Whoever "flew" in and out of our home heard Jay's powerful testimony.

In truth, Jay's ability to laugh in the face of death was a gift from God, too. It infused joy into our spirits.

About that same time, Jay was asked to speak again—this time at a worship service designed to meet the needs of church members seeking to recover from an addiction, emotional problem, or illness. Jay and I spoke at the July 2006 Recovery Service. There we were: Jay in his wheelchair and I by his side, holding the microphone. His speech was much slower and more deliberate by then.

As Jay shared his testimony of growing faith, he publicly expressed gratitude for all I did in the background as his caregiver. He inadvertently called me his "trophy wife," which brought down the house! People roared with laughter and applauded, as Jay glanced at me with a sheepish "oops" look on his face. He would explain later that he didn't mean it how it sounded, but by then, it was too late to recover what he had truly intended. The Recovery Service has never been the same.

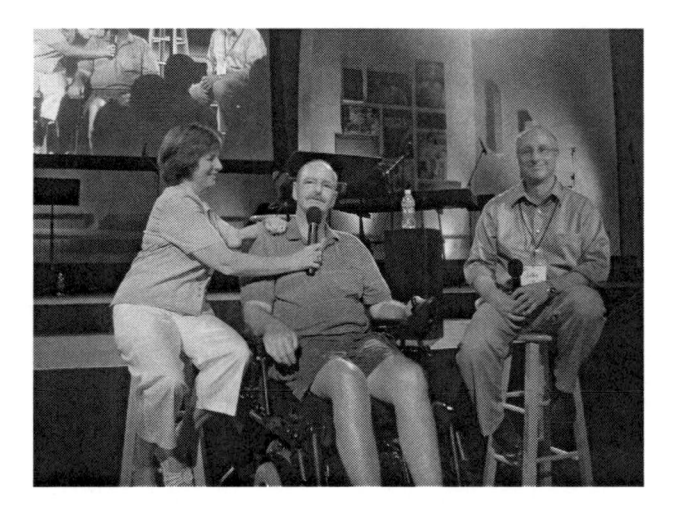

Jay describing my role as his caregiver to the body of believers at Ginghamsburg recovery service. John Jung, Jay's mentor and friend moderated.

I must mention that during the "trophy wife" hysteria we amassed that day at church, Jay announced to his audience he was being called to a public-speaking ministry. Little did Jay and I know that Chuck Cox, the county sheriff, was present in the audience. With his help, along with Prison Chaplain Mary Perry, Jay was almost immediately scheduled to speak twice at the Life Skills class of inmates at the county jail. Jay also recruited our associate pastor, Mike Bowie, and mentor, John Jung, to speak to the Life Skills class at the jail.

When Jay spoke to these men about his struggle with life and death issues, you could have heard the proverbial pin drop. He told the inmates, "Never give up, no matter how tough life's challenges are. God can use you right where you are."

> For I was hungry, and you fed me.
> I was thirsty and you gave me a drink.
> I was a stranger, and you invited me into your home.
> I was naked, and you gave me clothing.
> I was sick and you cared for me.
> I was in prison, and you visited me.
> —Matthew 25:35–36

At the conclusion of the Life Skills classes, Jay attended the inmates' graduation ceremony. He appeared on the local television news and received many accolades from those prisoners inspired by his speech. One young man drew and presented him with a lifelike color sketch of praying hands holding a cross. It bore the message, "You have been sent Angels to watch over you."

Many inmates wrote him thank-you notes for giving them courage and faith to face the future and to start again. Here are a few excerpts that flowed from the hearts of the young men:

Dear Mr. Jay Jordan, I know the Lord was using you to reach me in a way that I'll NEVER 4-get the rest of my lifetime. You spoke with much compassion and I deeply admired your integrity. It must have been much of a challenge for you to get in front of a bunch of strange men, not only men, but inmates. I am sure we will all remember and cherish your talk. I am sure it will inspire us the rest of our lifetimes.

Dear Mr. Jay Jordan, I would like to say thank you for the time and effort it took for you to come here … Your story was very touching and inspiring and moved me in a way that is unexplainable … I have met this guy (you) who is almost laid to rest, but yet you have such a positive attitude. You were willing to share your story with a group of confused individuals. I admire your courage, determination, and all faith in the Lord and the positive lifestyle of you and your family. I believe your testimony gave me the peace I was searching for all so many years in the past. I pray for you and your family every night.

Dear Jay, I thank you for coming and sharing with all of us in Life Skills. It broke me down inside; it draw tears from my face. I believe every word that you said to me. It was true stuff. It come out of your heart that I cry when we went back to our cell pod. I have to do the right things when I walk out of these walls, and to be a better person for myself and take the right way, not the wrong way. I just lost my father December 20, 2005. It has changed my life around. I keep looking out these windows looking up to the sky. I know my father is looking over me every day and night. I pray every day and night to wake up every morning to smile at life. Thank you and your family for coming out and sharing with us. I hope you will be around for loving God. I will pray for you and your wife and son. I started to get into the Bible more. I read a few more lines from Matthew 26 and understood a little better how Jesus' blood covered my sins ... Thank you for everything you said. God will be with you Jay. I love you.

Dear Jay, I want to thank you and your family from the bottom of my heart. You have truly touched my heart in a way no one could. You are a great inspiration. It's nice to see there is still love in this world. It does the heart good to know that a man in your condition can still think of others. I pray that I can take meeting you on through life (with me and that) it will let me be a better person. I think you are a Godly man who has more love and respect for mankind than anyone I ever met. Every day I will pray for you and your family for the rest of my life no matter how long or short it may be. I am a handyman by trade and if there is anything I can do for you or your family, please don't think twice about calling on me.

To Mr. Jay Jordan … You touched me with everything that came out of your mouth that day. You taught me a few things in our brief time that we talked. You let me in on some very important information such as: No matter how tough things get, never give up. Keep your head held high … I want to do good in life, such as be a good citizen, father, husband, brother, uncle, and all that. I know what I need to do to be that, thanks to you.

Everywhere—from Jay's bedside to the church to the county jail and yes, even over a game of checkers on the porch at the nearest Cracker Barrel—our journey with Christ through the valley of the shadow of death was being shared. There always seemed to be something to smile about, because Jay was making an eternal investment of love in others … despite his infirmity and our human frailties. We had once again found smiles and purpose in serving others: our saving grace.

CHAPTER TEN

COMING TO TERMS WITH DEATH

and the Sauerkraut Incident

Sometimes, when all else failed, we could laugh about something mundane. I guess that's what happens when living with impending death every day.

For instance, on the day after Jay's PEG tube was surgically inserted, two of his friends came to sit with Jay so I could go out to dinner with their wives. When we returned a couple of hours later, there was a strange car in the driveway. During the course of Jay's illness, the back door into our house remained unlocked, so I did not have to answer the door around the clock. People just let themselves in. Until that occasion, a stranger had never entered our home.

When we went inside, my friends and I met a woman we didn't recognize or know standing in my kitchen. Our three very sheepish-looking husbands, who began to confess their guilt, surrounded her. It turned out that Jay had experienced nausea, sweating, and general malaise after supper. The men sitting with Jay had called hospice, who sent a member of their staff, Debbie. She had come immediately to assess Jay's condition. By the time she had arrived, he was feeling better, she reported.

I asked Jay what he had eaten for dinner. Until then, no one had divulged that little secret. It seems that Jay ate a Reuben sandwich with french fries and drank a beer. They were afraid to tell the nurse … and us! If it hadn't struck all of us as so funny, and if I hadn't been so relieved that Jay was all right, I might not have bopped him "upside the head."

Beneath my feigned objections, I could understand. Jay was becoming less able to enjoy the sense of taste, because he couldn't swallow with ease. It was another ominous sign the disease was taking over.

A sad day of foreboding occurred when an aide took off Jay's wedding ring due to chronic edema. We put his ring on a chain, which he wore about his neck. Meanwhile, I tried everything to get him to let me feed him, but he refused to cooperate and began to eat less and less.

"My biggest fear," Jay once said, "is that I'm going to get to a place where I absolutely hate to be on this planet, because of the shape I'm in before God takes me home. When I lose my ability to eat, I'm going to be very unhappy."

Although Jay regretted being unable to do things for himself, I had to be careful not to baby him. For instance, one evening when I cradled his neck with a pillow and placed a crocheted shawl over his lap, he quipped, "Don't make me look like an invalid!"

We both chuckled, but I was scared, and so was he. I asked, "If your disease stopped progressing now, would you be happy?"

His reply was sad but certain. "No, there would be no quality of life."

I didn't blame him. It just seemed surreal to think of how far we had come—and yet, how far we still might have to go in dealing with this agonizing way of life … and Jay's departure. While he could still guide me, I began learning how to manage the financial records he kept online so that I could take over the monthly budget responsibilities. The number of accounts and passwords involved surprised me.

We spent almost every moment of every day together, and every day

I could see Jay losing ground. But when I would leave the house, he always rose to the occasion to tease me. As I excused myself to run errands, he told a newspaper reporter, who was interviewing him, "Katie spends most of the afternoons getting her hair done and going to Hobby Lobby."

We thought the end may come any time, because his lower left lung had collapsed. Antibiotics were administered, but he was so exhausted, his body didn't seem to be fighting off infection. With his breathing quite shallow, carbon dioxide was building up in his body, which caused him to doze and sleep around the clock.

Although he began to talk more and more about his final wishes, I think he held some thoughts to himself. It would take an extraordinary person at just the right time to bring his thoughts to the surface. On July 22, 2006, John Jung helped us begin to map out the funeral service (almost a full year before Jay would die). John was on the Ginghamsburg Church staff as director and psychologist for New Creation Counseling Center. Having trained Jay for lay pastor ministry, he had been a dear friend and mentor for years. John came at least once a week and always brought beer to share.

Once the dialogue was opened, ideas and desires began to flow. Jay began to think about who he would like to serve as pallbearers, as well as favorite Bible verses and songs. He commissioned me to go to the funeral home and discuss these and other matters with the staff. When I took along a picture of our selected gravestone, my emotions got the better of me. I was pulled aside by Velvet, who listened to me pour out my grief. She said something so affirming that it still provides comfort and healing for that overriding sense of guilt that I have battled. She said, "Few people touch us like you and Jay have done. It's God at work in you."

God, can you hear me?
Can you move him along or supply a miracle?
I can't see either of us staying in this state much longer.

I cringe in fear with things asked of me.
I'm so afraid I'll drop him, or not be able to move him.
I don't want him to be afraid of asking me for help.
I seem to cause him more physical torture when I try to help.
Lord, let us both do what is right and help us
open up to each other as never before.
I don't want to miss any opportunity to create memories.
Make him comfortable in this place, and not see this
house as a place he moved into to die.
Make it an oasis and not a trap to him.
I don't know how to help.
I love him and will be lost without him, but I will survive.

There were always some concerned friends who really didn't know what to do with our circumstances or us. Death frightens most, and I understand, because before Jay got sick, I didn't "do" death and dying either. Yet, whenever there was a need we didn't know how to handle, God would send us another mat carrier from the community.

On one occasion, Jay's temporary power chair was broken. Luke bought a soldering gun to try to repair it, but his attempts failed. In the meantime, we had decided to order a pizza for dinner. When the pizza delivery guy arrived with dinner in hand, Luke asked him if he knew how to solder metal. As a result, he came in and fixed Jay's chair.

On another evening, Jay had fallen out of his chair when I was transferring him from the bed. I couldn't get him up. I immediately thought of calling Jim Yardley, who had offered the night before to come when needed. So I phoned him, and Jim was there in ten minutes. Jay was lifted into his bed and after a little rest, into the chair.

Our faith grew when we saw such specific evidences of the supernatural touch of God. Although the healing we had prayed for hadn't happened, we had learned to place our entire emotional and spiritual dependence on His eternal resources. We began to imagine what Jay's homecoming in Heaven would be like. I was sure God would welcome Him with open arms and the affirmation, "Well done, my good and faithful servant."

But Jay's life wasn't over yet. He still harbored a few more important things to check off his bucket list.

Day by day, the Lord takes care of the innocent ...

—Psalm 37:18

CHAPTER ELEVEN

JAY LAST "WALK" AND LAST HURRAH

To Boldly Go Where No Terminally Ill Man Has Gone Before ...

With my instructions posted everywhere and the doors perpetually unlocked, our faithful army of mat carriers continued to come and go at will. The stimulation of having extra people on hand seemed to keep Jay's interest in life piqued, even as his body atrophied to dead weight.

Jay nicknamed everyone who came into our home to help us, and they all loved his creative, spunky outlook. There were hospital aides simply known as "Donut Girl" or "Mutt and Jeff" and friends known as "Pickles" Bailar or "The Church Ladies," Marcia and Donna. Depending on their personality, appearance, or caregiving role, names were assigned as though Jay were knighting his entire court. They loved it, and Jay loved them.

Although his body was paralyzed, Jay's will was never broken. His mind was still fertile (perhaps a bit too fertile for his own good) with plans and possibilities. His attitude of great expectations continued to amaze all who knew him, including his primary caregiver, who was still learning to be flexible—like a rubber band.

On September 10, 2006, another community opportunity for Jay to shine presented itself. Our Dayton Walk to Defeat ALS, sponsored by the ALS Association, was scheduled to raise awareness and funds for support services, such as respite care and home health equipment, as well as research. This would be our second walk since Jay was diagnosed.

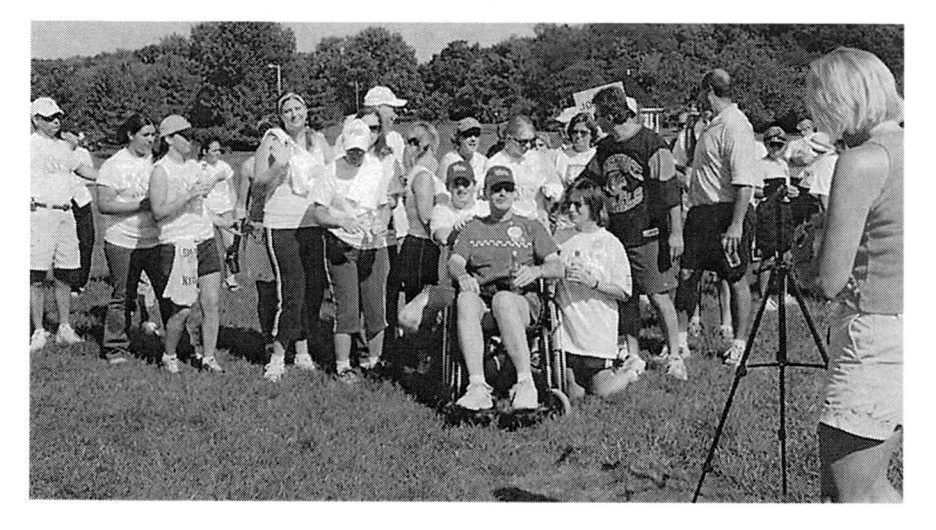

Jay and the ALS walk team

Because I was so involved in managing Jay's care and Jay could no longer use the phone and computer to recruit team members and sponsors, our friends Cheryl and Dave Jett chaired our 2006 walk team efforts. As the Jetts were preparing our team letter of appeal, Jay asked that one of his favorite quotes be placed at the top of the letter beside our picture.

The quote was passed to us through Bobette Borchardt, our friend with terminal cancer. Although the author of this quotation is unknown, it perfectly describes Jay's personality and spirit:

> My goal in this life's journey is not to arrive at the grave safely
> in a well-preserved body, but rather to skid in sideways, totally
> worn out, shouting ... "What a ride!"

Some of our church members got on board to help raise funds and mail copious letters of appeal. Our team grew by leaps and bounds under the Jetts' direction, and they used every resource at their disposal to round up as much support as possible. It seemed that Jay's positive attitude had won him a great following of supporters.

The week before the ALS Walk, Cheryl arranged for Luke and me to talk about Jay, ALS, and the event at Luke's high school alma mater, Troy Christian. We met with classes and showed the vignette Luke had recorded for a senior class project, based on the popular contemporary Christian song sung by Casting Crowns, "Praise You in this Storm, by Mark Hall and Bernie Herms.

And I'll praise you in this storm
and I will lift my hands
for You are who You are
no matter where I am.

Set to the music of this song, our melancholy son is seen as he walks alone, surrounded by stormy nature's beauty. He silently ponders the reality of his father's illness and ultimate loss, and yields his grief to God. As a result of the presentation, students were moved to action and signed up to be on our Journey for Jay team.

However, on the Thursday night before Sunday's ALS Walk, Jay had to be admitted to the inpatient unit at Dayton Hospice with an uncontrolled fever of 103 degrees. When those attending him advised keeping him at hospice for a few days, it appeared he would miss the walk.

The doctors didn't realize they were dealing with a strong-willed child. He wasn't about to miss the ALS Walk! In truth, he didn't allow himself to stay downhearted about his disease. He was too busy keeping us both in the mainstream of life.

So, at Jay's insistence, we asked permission to spring him from hospice on Sunday morning just in time to attend the event. I promised we would return immediately following the walk, so he could continue his inpatient care until the doctors deemed him well enough to go home. The attending physician and staff just looked at us and shook their heads. They flatly informed us that, due to policy, if Jay left the premises, he would have to be discharged. Despite our better judgment, Jay's determination won out. So, Luke and I bathed and dressed him at the very last minute, and he was front and center, in time to meet his adoring public at the walk.

The day was quite festive, with music, information booths, food galore, and even clowns making balloon animals for all the young people involved. Troy Christian School sent a busload of students, who rallied around Jay like fans to a celebrity. The Journey for Jay team was obviously a spirited bunch, especially since Luke and his friends sported silly balloon hats and cheered us with the exuberance only teenagers can demonstrate. Naturally, Luke and his friends sprinted the walk and finished long before anyone else! With the vigilance of a mother bear guarding her cub, I limited Jay to one symbolic lap around the track before we departed for home.

By late fall of 2006, Jay was visibly slowing down, but he had one final mission he wanted to accomplish. I might have expected it to be next to impossible, and it was. All the more reason Jay insisted on making it happen.

His dream? To take one last flight as a passenger—in a fighter jet that would take him soaring into the wild blue yonder, upside down, spiraling. The works!

Sometimes I think I deserved to have a nervous breakdown. This was one of those times. We who heard this preposterous notion just shook our heads and said, "It'll never happen." Jay's body was as limp and lifeless as a bowl of gelatin. There was no feasible way he could survive fast-paced, aerobatic maneuvers like a Blue Angel, much less get into the plane.

I've learned never to say "never," because it turned out that Jay and God were in cahoots on this little scheme. Everyone entering our home heard about Jay's last wish. The message gradually filtered into the community.

For example, our friend David Jett told his professional colleagues at American Airlines. They were impressed with Jay and his dream. Someone said they knew a pilot from another airline who owned an

Italian fighter trainer, a distinctive, butterfly-tail jet called the Fouga CM-170 Magister. The pilot was contacted and was more than agreeable to arrange a flight for Jay—if the logistics related to Jay's condition could be managed.

From there, things started to happen. The Sidney Fire Department agreed to provide an emergency medical rescue harness to attach to Jay's limp body, so he could be placed into the cockpit. Meanwhile, Piqua Steel committed the manpower and crane that would lift Jay into his seat behind the pilot.

Of course, Pilot John (last name withheld to protect the guilty!) provided his time, expertise, and gear for his unique passenger. So many people were ultimately involved in making Jay's last wish come true that remembering this experience gives me goose bumps. I can only imagine this meant absolutely everything to a dying man with a passion for flight and adventure.

After some pensive moments related to weather delays, Jay was cleared for takeoff on the partly cloudy, chilly morning of December 11, 2006. He had more attendants than the King of England, as they fussed over every detail of his well-being and preparation for the flight. With helmet, communication gear, protective vest, and harness in place, Jay was ready. The magic moment had finally arrived, and he was hoisted by crane into the jet's passenger seat behind the pilot. I must applaud all involved in this most daring caper for their excellent performance and attention to safety. After all, that was my husband dangling above that jet on a hook!

Jay was a satisfied customer as he sat in position. I reached up to do a last-minute security check and tucked a neck pillow in place. Like a girlfriend bidding her handsome young military hero off to battle, I gave him a kiss good-bye. He would have passed for a star from the movie *Top Gun* to anyone who hadn't witnessed the acrobatics and engineering of preparing Jay for flight.

Since Jay could barely speak, he and the pilot exchanged some facial expressions that served as their communication, and they took to the skies. Luke recorded the entire process, and we onlookers stood by and froze to death. But it was an awe-inspiring spectacle to behold, as the jet soared into the heavens with a beautiful, passionate, fun-loving dreamer on board. I'm not sure I breathed the entire time they were airborne.

It was clear all our teamwork and angst paid off, when the jet landed and the cockpit door opened. With everyone applauding and the pilot giving a thumbs up, there was Jay, blue eyes wide and smile beaming. His only lament to me later was, "We didn't turn upside down!"

Forever and Beyond
Lyrics and Music by
Sam Mizell and Matthew West;

If I could reach, reach above the clouds
Higher than the rain could find me
And I would reach, reach beyond the stars
Into a place where love will last forever and beyond

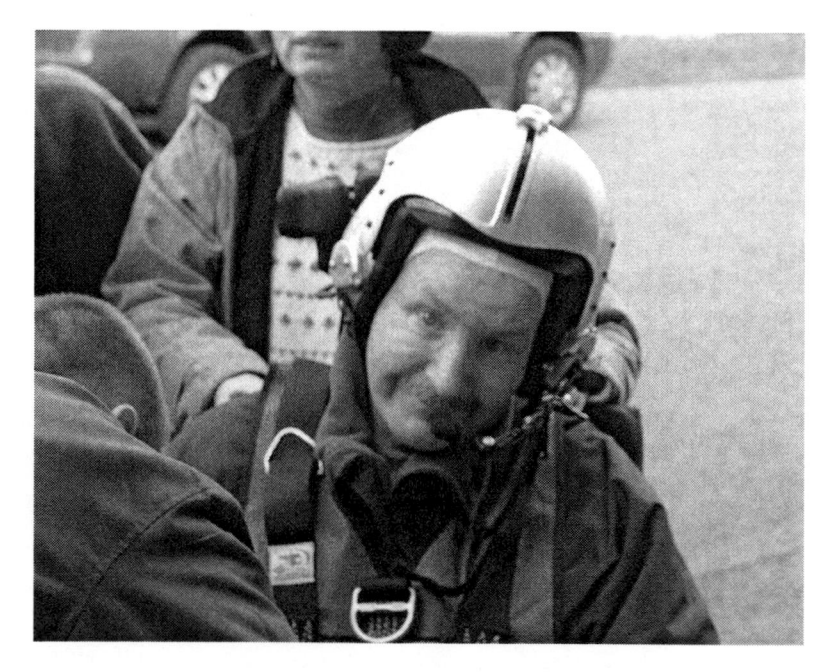

preparing for his last earthly flight

CHAPTER TWELVE

FINAL CELEBRATIONS ...

Fueled by "A Different Kind of Love"

After Jay's flight, his demeanor mellowed and retired from earthly ambition. With his voice faltering, the speaking ministry that had exponentially given him purpose sadly came to an end. He seemed resigned to sit at home and wait for a visitor, Night Angel, or aide from hospice to appear. He would tease, cajole, and dub them with some silly name, and all would be well for a while. Every guest and mat carrier who entered our home restored his bright smile.

Jay's last Christmas season (2006), was bittersweet and beautifully filled with laughter and the comfort of friends and family. Although he would have six more months to live, his health was clearly unstable. I believe he might have given into death sooner had his life not been prolonged and enriched by the presence of our loving mat carriers. Whatever the time frame, we all were determined to make every day count. Until the very month Jay died, celebrations abounded.

For Christmas, our friends creatively gifted us with written word and deeds, which transcended the trappings of the season. Their thoughtfulness resonated with our heart's cries. I kept notes they gave us, which are now tucked into my scrapbooks.

One of these messages announced a very special gift—a brick on a

Veterans Memorial Walk—sent from Jeff and Bobette Borchardt, even as they coped with Bobette's terminal cancer. Her handwritten note is worth a mint of gold:

> To Our Dear Sweet Brother,
> You know how we wanted to be buried next to each other and that couldn't be worked out ... So we wanted to do something special for you and your family for Christmas. You and Jeff will be permanently next to each other, memorialized at the Veterans Memorial Wall in Riverside Cemetery. The Memorial was established to honor all veterans who have served or who are now serving in the Armed Forces for the preservation of freedom throughout the world. The engraved bricks will be laid this spring, and we will be notified of their exact location. Yours will read:
>
>
>
> E. W. "Jay" Jordan
> Vietnam War
> May 1970–May 1971
>
>

Another Christmas message came from Alan and Pamela Bailar, who announced, "A donation has been made in your name to the Ginghamsburg Church Love Fund" (which helps the needy in our community).

Millie Arnold of Jackson Center, Ohio, presented a cheerful, hand-sewn holiday coverlet. Janice offered the gift of prayer: "Jay, thinking of you every day. I am remembering you in my prayers."

When our three children arrived home for the holidays, so did their friends from the area. Overhearing the jovial banter lightened our moods and brought the house to life. Together, we decorated the Christmas tree, while Jay watched us at our silliest. We hung all our Christmas cards, as well as ornaments and twinkle lights, on the branches of the Christmas tree. My mother and sister came down from Lima, Ohio, to enjoy part of the holiday with us. We must have taken a zillion and one photographs, and Jay sipped his holiday cheer (beer) through a straw.

On New Year's Eve, 2006, our friends from the Sowers and Reapers cell group planned for Pastor Mike Bowie to serve communion at our home. A funny side-note occurred when Mike locked his keys inside his house and had to hitch a ride to our house with another church staff member. Although he ran a bit late, he administered the bread and the wine, representing Christ's body and blood, and read Jay's requested passage of Scripture:

> I assure you, anyone who believes in me already has eternal life.
> Yes, I am the bread of life!
> Your ancestors ate manna in the wilderness, but they all died.
> However, the bread from heaven gives eternal
> life to everyone who eats it.
> I am the living bread that came down out of heaven.
> Anyone who eats this bread will live forever;
> This is my flesh, offered so the world may live.
> Then the people began arguing with
> each other about what he meant.
> "How can this man give us his flesh to eat?" they asked.
> So Jesus said again, "I assure you,
> Unless you eat the flesh of the Son of Man and drink His blood,
> You cannot have eternal life within you."
> —John 6:47–53

Receiving Holy Communion at church can be a most significant event, but experiencing it in our living room with friends, who were willing to forge the unknown "valley of the shadow of death" experiences with us, was especially meaningful. Following the Scripture reading, Mike Bowie and John Jung anointed all those present with oil, and we sang John Newton's hymn "Amazing Grace":

> *Amazing Grace, how sweet the sound,*
> *That saved a wretch like me.*
> *I once was lost but now am found,*
> *Was blind, but now I see.*

T'was Grace that taught my heart to fear.
And Grace, my fears relieved.
How precious did that Grace appear
The hour I first believed.

Through many dangers, toils and snares
I have already come;
'Tis Grace that brought me safe thus far
and Grace will lead me home.

When we've been here ten thousand years
Bright shining as the sun.
We've no less days to sing God's praise
Than when we've first begun.

Afterward, Pamela "Pickles" Bailar called me into the guest bathroom. She reported the toilet was broken. I knew nothing about how to repair a toilet. As luck would have it, Reed Sevitts appeared, as if by magic. The three of us had a long, lively discussion about what might be wrong with the toilet, and Reed checked the tank for potential issues. In the end, the great ceramic bowl seemed to be working just fine. I was beginning to grow suspicious.

When I came out, balloons and a sprawling pile of colorfully packaged gifts had taken over the living room. The kitchen had been transformed into a buffet. "The Church Ladies"—Marcia Niswonger and Donna Sevitts—had planned a surprise birthday party for me. Everyone present was in on the surprise!

Everyone around the room lifted a glass and proposed toasts. A few flying monkeys were released, but you would have had to be there to totally understand. Jim Dean, a loyal leader of the Recovery Service and the twelve-step program, ironically assisted Jay with a New Year's Eve toast.

I had never felt so affirmed and loved. Thanks to our friends, 2007 was launched with vision and purpose. This was the year Jay would move from this life to the next, but we were not afraid due to the love and thoughtfulness of our mat carriers.

Saturday Night Live

Move over, Jay Leno. For several months, Alan and Pamela "Pickles" Bailar had been joining us for church. They first came to our house, and we would get Jay ready, and off we would go. Alan drove and parked the van, and accompanied us home after the service. In addition, we rotated restaurants for carry-out. We enjoyed commiserating over dinner and wine with a daily devotional study of Oswald Chambers.

Marcia and Gary Niswonger eventually joined us. Marcia, being the event planner that she is, began cooking dinner for the six of us. As the weather grew colder, Jay and I could no longer attend worship at church. But because of our friends' creative efforts, we benefited from the fellowship of our own version of *Saturday Night Live*.

Thank you, friends.

~~~

Also in January, our home health agency informed us of a policy change that affected us: they would no longer provide care to private-pay patients. We were given three months to find another agency.

We decided on American Nursing, who sent us Valerie, who Jay dubbed "Cover Girl"; Debbie "the Informer"; and Lisa, "the Bronzed Beauty." These three ladies joined our squadron of caregivers, including Alicia, who Jay named "NASCAR Nurse," and others who came to us through staffing agencies to cover Sunday shifts. While Jay could still enjoy tasting food, some of his attendants would bring carry-out food—everything from pizza to Bourbon Street chicken. These were competent aides who kept Jay company as well as saw to his health-care needs.

On the eve of Valentine's Day 2007, our aides phoned to say they were snowed in and couldn't get out of their driveways to report to work.

After Jay fell asleep, I asked God for strength to get through the next day, which would be Day 2 of caring for Jay by myself.

That morning, bathing and dressing took longer than usual. I had not gotten a chance to clean up the bathroom or the bedroom. I felt my time was best served by attending Jay.

While we were eating lunch, David Jett walked in, assessed the situation, and recruited his wife, Cheryl, to come right over. While David and daughter Hannah went to the store for dinner preparations, Cheryl cleaned, changed the bed, and took care of laundry duties. Meanwhile, I was instructed to shower and go to bed. It was heavenly.

David and Hannah returned with a feast! Later, for dinner, we had assorted fish, potatoes, watermelon, asparagus, and poppy seed muffins. Cheryl fed Jay. They came just when we needed them most. God had heard and answered my prayer with Jett family strength.

When I returned to the family room later, a card was face up on the table. It said:

> You have a God who hears you,
> the power of love behind you,
> the Holy spirit within you,
> and all of heaven ahead of you.
> —Max Lucado

For Valentine's Day, I had entered a contest sponsored by KLove Radio. Mark Schultz, a Christian singer, was going to write a Valentine's song from one love story. Although mine didn't win, Jay was touched by my story about us and even admitted my writing had improved!

I wrote "A Different Kind of Love," in which I expressed,

> This Valentine's Day will be very special for us. Without a miracle, it will be our last. We don't know for sure when that day will come. Jay has no use of his arms or legs and needs

all his basic care performed for him. We haven't been able to hug each other for over a year. His voice is almost gone, and "I love you" has become a whisper. Our days are spent sitting side by side with my holding his hand and reading to him from our devotionals and the Bible. Gone are the dinners out, the flowers, and candy. In their place is the hope for an eternal life and the longing for those things yet to be seen.

> *Jay's purpose?*
> *To show others how to live while dying.*
> *Mine?*
> *To be there with this wonderful man until death parts us.*

Our next celebration was spawned from the planning of the Church Ladies. They gained my prior approval for an open house in honor of Jay's fifty-seventh birthday. It was scheduled for February 18, from 2 to 5 p.m., and remained a secret until that morning, when we opted to put shoes instead of slippers on Jay. He guessed something was up.

With the help of our cell group friends, Marcia and Donna oversaw all decorations, invitations, food, room arrangements, and procuring live music. Jay received over sixty cards, and many old acquaintances were renewed. Handwritten notes inside the cards informed Jay how much his life and journey meant to each person.

During the open house, Paul Jones and Donnie Reis performed contemporary Christian music. Helium balloons, thousands it seemed, were filled (and got tangled up) in our living room, curly ribbons and all. "Queen Bee" Marcia and Pamela "the French Maid" Bailar served cake with candles and punch. Jay enjoyed greeting his guests from his easy chair, beneath a blanket. Due to his limitations, Marcia and I blew out his candles, but he made his own wish.

In addition, Jay's family came from Kentucky, along with my family members and friends. Bobette was able to be with us, as were lots of friends from out of town. He later reflected on how touched and honored he felt that so many people would stop by to see him.

A LIMERICK

From a Friend Who Doesn't Know His
Iambic Pentameter from a Hole in the Ground
—Reed Sevitts-

There once was a fellow from Kentucky
Whose life wasn't always so ducky
His sins of the past,
Forgiven at last
Has made him blessed and lucky.

This fella from Flemingsburg, Jay,
He's got it soft every day
He's fluffed, buffed, and fed
Then tucked into bed
While those around him do pray.

His life is exciting you'll agree
Ask plaintiffs one, two, or three.
Rides in helicopters and jets
Break him out in cold sweats
And causes him to release pee

You see, Jay, we love you at best.
This fun is poked at you in jest.
Though we clown around
When it's time to get down
We all realize we are blessed

We celebrate this day of your birth.
The food will increase our girth.
We'll exclaim quite bold
My God, man, you're old
But our friendship is the true worth.

When the glorious party came to an end, the party planners whisked everything away, as though it never happened. All evidence was discarded. Alan Bailar swept the hardwood floors to a glorious finish. In these more festive moments shared with friends, we gained strength and courage for whatever challenge was around the next bend.

~~~

Now, you might think we let down our guard for the Grim Reaper after Jay's birthday party, but you are wrong. What could possibly trump such a celebration but a little March Madness!

March Madness

Sheriff Charles Cox had been trying for a month of Saturdays to pin a DUI on Jay under suspicion only. His charge was based on erratic driving of a wheelchair. The evidence involved numerous "dings" on the walls and door facings of the house, accompanied by uncontrollable laughter.

One Saturday night, he arrived to find a staged collection of empty beer bottles lined up on Jay's medicine table. Being the ever-vigilant officer of the law that he was, he said nothing. Several days later, we received an authentic ticket of violation via the US Postal Service, stating the conditions of our home and ordering us to appear before the sheriff on March 30, 2007.

Of course, we immediately hired an "attorney," or at least borrowed the letterhead. We responded in a timely manner to the charges. The following letter was sent in rebuttal:

Dear Sir or Madam,

We have been retained by Eldon W. Jordan, et al. in the matter concerning said ticket issued 3/9/07. It has herewith been brought to our attention that Mr. Jordan is an alleged party involved in a DUI. It is so noted on the said document that the party of the first part was operating a vehicle at night on a brick pavement under extremely hazardous conditions. The defendant, upon viewing said ticket, cried out, "I've been framed!"

At no time did you indicate that a field sobriety Breathalyzer test or radar detection was utilized in the proper manner as set forth in the penal code of Sheriffs USA. In addition to these above rebuttals, we question the medical health of the arresting officer. Please cease and desist immediately, or we will bring an ALSHC (ALS harassment charge) against your department and suggest a disciplinary hearing among your peers. This might also involve strip stripping.

Sincerely,
XXXXXXX

In response to the letter, we were then instructed to bribe the sheriff with a dozen donuts (minus the one Luke ate) and call it even. Jay got such a kick out of this prank that I believe it possibly bought him another week or two of life!

~~~

In April, Jay, clad in shorts and T-shirt and coated with sunscreen, was wheeled onto the patio for his first sunbath of the year. By May, he was bundled under quilted blankets, while everyone else was in short sleeves to stroll the grounds.

Also in April, crisis care nurses came to help me for a full week when Jay had pneumonia. As his dad was resting in his easy chair, Luke produced a baby bunny from the yard to show his father.

In those final months, all modesty was set aside when one of our Night Angels, Dancing Queen Beth Thoele, a former high school standout cheerleader, invented and demonstrated the "elimination cheer" to help Jay with his most challenging bodily functions. Believe me, we all cheered when Jay was successful!

Until the last possible moment, all of us rallied about Jay to give him the greatest send-off we possibly could. We kept him rallied until his body began to shut down. Then, we tried to keep him comforted as well as comfortable. I prayed for sweet release for my precious husband. He was ready to go. I couldn't think about how his departure would affect me until after I saw him to Heaven's gate.

CHAPTER THIRTEEN

HOMECOMING

Journal Entries from the Last Month of Jay's Life

May 28, 2007—Jay's body is really giving out … We put him in his recliner. and he was asleep in 20 minutes after I read. He stayed asleep until 8:30. I fed him ice. Deb and Jim put him to bed. I read to him, and he was asleep again by 10:15. No dinner. No hunger. No words. Just sleep. I prayed God would be merciful and take him, but I feel my prayers were selfish and not right. I feel so inadequate.

May 30, 2007—I feel productive today. I had a plan, and things went smoothly. Last night, David Jett was over, and Jay asked him to be a pallbearer. David asked me in front of Jay if I planned to stay in the house. He asked Jay other death questions, but I left the room.

We have a new nightly ritual. I read Jay to sleep. He forces himself awake, so I will continue. He told Kathy I had a beautiful reading voice. I told him I loved him, and he didn't say it back.

May 31, 2007—I'm sitting here watching Jay sleep. I just finished reading the Max Lucado book *Six Hours One Friday*. He slept through most of it, but I did it mostly for me. Now I'm trying to get myself onto my knees to ask for release from his bondage.

I talked to Judie, Dr. Cass, John, and Reid, and all but Reid felt the time was near. Jay voiced he wanted to wait on God and not help it along with the medications that hospice can provide to ease his suffering… Jay doesn't make much sense when I ask him what he wants … Jay will ask Jim Meyer (along with David Jett) to be his pallbearers. I want to add Scott Rowlett if he doesn't. I told John and Reed that I don't know how much more of this I can take. I can't understand him, and it is exhausting to figure out what he wants.

I worry about who will be there for me down the road? Will I be alone or face another life like I did after the divorce? Too much fear, as Lucado says. There should only be celebration and singing. I want to sing. I want to celebrate! I want to know that he is home and dancing with the angels, healthy and worshipping constantly … I want peace!

> *God please hear our prayers.*
> *I don't want to be selfish.*
> *But how long must we wait?*

June 4 2007—Jay's confusion is growing. Last night, we put him to bed. Then he asked us if we were getting ready to put him on the toilet, where he wanted to be. Dr. Cass of hospice wants morphine around the clock. I told her she had to tell Jay that. Jay rarely acknowledges people—except Deb Meyer. We had the Saturday night crowd over, and I spoon-fed some daiquiri. He seemed to enjoy it. I feel I need to lay with him. I just can't make myself do it.

Mom came down, and I cried in front of her about my disappointment in our friend backing away. She cried, too. She has the same problem. I pray I can be there for people, as they need me physically as well as with cards/notes, etc. No one knows what to say or do. I have never felt so helpless in all my life. So out of control.

June 5, 2007—I stayed home today, because Dr. Cass and Vicky were here. Meds were changed. Vicky told me he is in transition. We have weeks remaining. I don't think so. Everyone that comes sees change. I see them daily.

Today he slept from 2 until 8:20 p.m. Ate a Popsicle, a half-can food, and ce. He coughs constantly and looks waxy. Vicky cried, as did I. I feel I need to be here and not leave, but it seems too much of a deathwatch.

I will continue to praise you, Lord. I ask you to take him to be with you.

June 6, 2007—I feel the urgency of writing daily. I went out for the day, and when I came home, Kelly had done her own thing with meds. Jay only slept fitfully for two hours. His breathing was labored. I gave him an ice and some supplement, and we spent an hour on the toilet with no success ... Luke came over, and I told him about Dad. He called Matt for me. I have no idea who'll call Sarah. Jay's skin is waxy, and his speech is unintelligible. I read to him tonight—more for me. I read about grief and how it never leaves, because the cause of the grief can never return to be repaired.

I have enjoyed this little book so much. I wish I could make Jay feel better. I feel important ... got a card from Vicky and talked to Laura, Bajus, and Jeff today.

Sunday, June 9—The Gulleys came down, and Sandy and I went to lunch. Jay slept from 11:30 to 8:00 and missed their whole visit. The night before it was 1 to 9. Saturday, I stayed home except to go to church as we were out. I asked Pamela and Alan to come over, because I am getting more fearful being home alone at night. John came over Friday night ... and I asked about upping the morphine. I wanted to know if God would forgive me, or if I would be full of guilt. John thought not, as Jay wanted to go.

Last night, I got up due to elbow pain, need for juice, need for supplement ... Tonight, it's moaning and the BiPAP alarm is ringing. I took it off and put him on oxygen. I managed to see 30 minutes of Luke's ball game. I feel pulled apart right now. I am feeling myself splitting into pieces. I need help, and I don't know where to turn. I don't feel abandoned by God. He's sent me the Bailars, Beth, and most recently, Sherry Fisher. I want a Ouiji board, a crystal ball, and an inside scoop ...

June 12, 2007—Last night, I slept from midnight until 7:00-ish. Jay is asking more and more for ice and drinks. Last night, I couldn't get him awake at 9, when the Meyers came to put him to bed. Deb was upset with Jay's unresponsiveness. He said the BiPAP didn't work last night …

Today I saw Dr. Nash. I lost three pounds and BP was 106/64! I sat in the sun in Tipp and ran into Amie Watson. She wants to come sing to Jay on Friday.

Then I went to UVMC and got a hug from Don, one of our former UVMC aides. He likes his jobs! Today, Jay has been awake and needful. I just can't understand him, which is so frustrating. Last night, I hit the floor on my knees, asking God for an end to this trial, guidance as to how to handle his needs. As usual, I didn't hear Him respond, because I talked.

However … when Amie reminded me that Jay had said August, I panicked at the thought of six more weeks. I hate to feel that way. I've been sitting here, trying to put into small sentences what Pamela means to me.

June 13, 2007—The day started with phone calls. It was the morning nursing staff saying Lisa had called off from work, and they couldn't find any replacement. I started Jay's meds, food, and paraphernalia removal. Then Lisa walked in! Go figure! They got him on the pot, and he started coughing. Temp was 99.5, pulse 109, blood pressure 90/64. I called hospice. We were suctioning. Vicky said he didn't qualify for hospice crisis care. She read her papers and changed her mind … started crisis care. Jay coughed all day—productive but can't get it up. I asked him many ways about antibiotic. I don't want to give it to him, but he said yes. Months ago, he didn't want it. I called Luke, Mom, Matt, talked to Sarah and my sister Betsy, Pamela, and Sarah. Sarah offered to come home. I told her not right now.

Janet came back tonight, as did Beth! Luke ordered pizza. I decided tonight I could no longer be at home alone at night by myself. I feel so scared and alone.

I told Cheryl that the worst of ALS and the best was the time to plan, yet these past two months of watching him die have been agonizing. There has been no dialogue. No one can prepare you for the pain of watching and not being able to stop the suffering. I kissed him tonight and told him again that when God was ready for him, I was ready to release him. I want him dancing with the angels.

June 16—I can't believe the stress of the past few days. I didn't think I had so many tears in me. Janet has been here Wednesday–Thursday and Saturday night. God answers prayers. Our hospice day help hasn't given him meds. I don't understand why. Matt flew in for a day; Betsy was here, Luke and I went to church. John Jung came over yesterday and called today. Mike Bowie called yesterday and prayed over the phone with me.

Pamela has been with me Friday and tonight. I feel like tonight is the night. We moved his bed to the kitchen due to his anxiety about being alone. As of now, he hasn't calmed down. His pulse is up, as is his blood pressure. He is so stressed.

He sobbed talking to Alan, Pamela, Lynne and Chuck, the boys, and me. Everyone is saying good-bye. As Mike's sermon said, "I am in pain, but it's only through pain that we can be of use to others."

June 22—Friday. I'm surprised I know what day it is. It is going to be hard to describe the past few days, but I will try with objectivity and as little anger as I can muster. As I write this, we have been giving Jay round-the-clock meds every two hours to keep him asleep. When he wakes, his anxiety goes sky-high and he coughs. We can't suction due to the thickness and jaw clenching. Crisis care stayed through Wednesday.

Wednesday, Jay asked to go to hospice. I tried to talk him out of it, because I knew he wanted to go there to die, but he was adamant. We started calling friends to accompany us on the ambulance ride to hospice of Dayton … John Jung, the Bailars, Gulleys, and Reid.

After much discussion, hospice sent us home … I realized that God was still working through Jay. I know how much he didn't want to go there, and I feel he was making the ultimate sacrifice and allowing sedation to take the burden off me.

Wednesday night/Thursday morning—he woke up, and Sandy tried to help me get his mouth open. Jay asked, "Why did you do this to me?" when he realized he was home. It took six hours to calm him down. I called a hospice nurse, and she helped navigate the system. She got the drugs straightened out, and morphine medications can be administered every two hours to ease Jay's pain.

Hospice was to reinstate crisis care, and they couldn't find anyone, so I called Deb Meyer, and she took the night shift. Jay's temp continued upward. I called hospice and informed them what we were doing. I reported that I couldn't suction due to Jay's clenched jaw, so they sent a nurse (Debbie Rose). Debbie made sure we had a plan to increase drugs if needed today to prevent the breakthroughs. I've never felt so tired as I do now. I can't stand watching his irregular breathing, but I'm here for him. We've had more prayers around him lately. All wishing him a trip to be with Christ.

June 24—It's Sunday, and another very restless night. On Saturday a.m., Jay's breathing changed to short gasps that gurgled. He looked like he was working so hard to breathe. Pulse kept climbing. Blood pressure dropped. The nurse said we should expect an early morning death. We were expecting it, but he leveled out, and it didn't come.

Yesterday, we kept visitors to a minimum, but Cheryl, John and Deb were over. Signs are down. I talked to him, and once, I thought he raised his eyebrow. We took turns watching, but his breathing was so gross it was hard to stay near him.

It rained, so we sat with blankets on the front porch rockers. We had prayer and singing celebration. The Meyerses and Bailars were over. We prayed and then sang "Amazing Grace." Conrad and Gracie Jett downloaded Jay's song "There Is a Redeemer," and we played it. I prayed out loud, as did Pamela, Jim. It was a party—a send-off.

Alan has been in and out, running errands. Keeping us supplied. We've eaten well and talked. Dinner last night was great. We laughed at the kids' antics. They were in rare form. Tipper actually tried to jump on Jay's bed! She knows the situation. Lots of calls and offers to help. Nothing to do.

Alan, Kelly, and I moved equipment around to the garage and car for removal from the house. Pamela and I got his burial clothes ready for him. The chain and ring will be the last things off of him. It means the most.

Sometime either Friday or Thursday … Gary and Melissa Cairns came over and again we prayed over Jay. That was when we heard his lungs fill up and rattle. I was glad they came. They have been so silent, and it made me feel better.

June 26, 2007—Tuesday—The coma continues. Hospice pulled out of crisis care yesterday, because they said Jay was "stable" and could be managed by family and friends. Luke stayed up all night to administer the medications and care. Pamela, Kelly, and I took care of the days and evenings.

I did send Pamela home today (but she's coming back to spend the nights with me). I am enjoying sitting here quietly and feel less guilty, because she is getting things done she needs to do.

Luke moved in and stopped working. He spent last night caulking, sanding, and painting in our bath and bedroom.

Matt was here this weekend and livened things up. Pamela and Alan continue to be angels for us. I keep asking God why He is letting Jay linger. I get no answer. Jay made the ultimate sacrifice when he asked to go to hospice to die—to try to remove this cross from me. I think that's what precipitated his words to me Thursday—"Why did you do this to me?" Probably meaning, "Why am I back home? Why am I not in Heaven?"

I continue to talk to him, read him the Twenty-Third Psalm, whisper memories, and tell him to go home.

God, teach me to ask for what I want. Jay's peaceful passing from this earth.
How long, my Father? How long?

June 27, 2007—Pamela and Marcia convinced me to go out to lunch. I felt myself becoming more agitated and kept glancing at my cell phone. I noticed that I had missed a call from home. When I called Kelly, she insisted that she had not called, but that I might want to go home, as Jay's breathing had changed. As I was driving, I called Luke, who met me there. Tipper was trying unsuccessfully to jump on Jay's bed. Luke placed her up there, first beside his dad and then on his chest. I took Jay's hand and stroked it down Tipper's head as he had done himself so many times. Once this last task was completed, he took his last breath.

2:15 p.m.—Homecoming.

> The Lord's loved ones are precious to Him;
> It grieves Him when they die.
> —Psalm 116:15

CHAPTER FOURTEEN

WHAT A RIDE!

Friends Remember ...

*My goal in this life's journey
is not to arrive at the grave safely in a well-preserved body,
but rather, to skid in sideways, totally worn out,
Shouting, "What a ride!"*

Indeed, right up to the very end, Jay lived his life abundantly, completely worn out and skidding into Heaven sideways. I can only imagine that he was whooping, skipping, shouting, "What a ride!" as he met the saints.

Relief washed over those of us present at the end of Jay's battle with ALS. Even our dog, Tipper, was clearly satisfied his struggle to breathe was finally over.

Clamor and confusion soon ensued over who had the authority to pronounce him dead. Jay's requested DNR (do not resuscitate) order was present at the time of his passing. However, since hospice staff had ended its home crisis care three days before, no one from that agency was present to witness his death. We called 9-1-1, which notified emergency medical and local law enforcement officials. Hospice informed us the protocol would have been to notify its staff first.

From my perspective, Shakespeare had it right. These "important" details were much ado about nothing. It seemed futile as to whether hospice or the officers present pronounced Jay's time of death. A gathering group of representatives waited with Luke, Pamela, and me for a total of three hours until hospice staff arrived. In the interim, circumstances were upsetting, but I kept thinking, *This too shall pass.* I was comforted in knowing that Jay was in the presence of His Savior.

In the days that followed, I tried to thank everyone who had been there for Jay and me during our time of need. I will forever be grateful for each of them, but would cite Pamela Bailar's presence during the final days of Jay's life as being of specific support to me, the caregiver. After Jay became comatose, she stayed each night so that I wouldn't be afraid. When he died, Pamela continued her support and presence, informing our ministers and those dearest to us and helping me field the challenges at hand.

As our family received friends at the funeral home that Friday evening, we never managed to form a visitation line. I found myself working the room, talking with and thanking everyone. When Pamela and I talked with Jay's longtime STNA, Kelly, she said Jay's life example had shown her the true nature of Christ. As a result, she committed her life to Jesus Christ. It was a joy to share with Kelly that her choice to become a follower of Jesus Christ had been Jay's dying hope. It was a tearful, happy victory resulting from Jay's battle with ALS.

Meanwhile, Jay's video vignette recordings played, fascinating all that attended. I remember Bill Duff, church staff member, declaring, "Jay was the DNA of our church." What a tribute!

At Jay's funeral, Pachelbel's "Canon in D" was played. Always a favorite of our family, it was the instrumental piece that had lullabied Luke in utero, labor, and delivery. Its lilting, beautiful repetition later calmed him as a young child, when we would wind up his musical teddy bear at the first sign of tears washing down his freckled cheeks. Now, at Jay's funeral, the song once again worked its comforting, calming magic on all our hearts.

I believe there were a lot of people close to Jay who could have done a remarkable job eulogizing him, but several admitted they would have broken down in tears in the middle of it and elected not to take that risk. Two of Jay's cronies, David Jett and Reed Sevitts, paid tribute to the man, drawing laughter as well as tears. Here are a few highlights:

Excerpts of the Eulogy by David Jett

I once knew a man called Bojangles, and he talked to me! I did not have the pleasure of knowing Jay before his ALS diagnosis. We met at our sons' graduation and quickly became close friends over the next two years.

Many times, I asked Jay if God had revealed His vision [of how Jay's life would turn out]. His answer was always that God would take him to the lowest possible place and then build his body back anew, as though he were born again. Now, being the literalist that I can be, I set out praying specifically for healing to occur.

As time passed, Jay's disease progressed, yet he seemed to embrace those changes. I never once heard him complain about the cup he was asked to endure. Not once ... What a testimony for me ... I have been truly blessed to have known Jay Jordan. His faith story made my [spiritual] roots grow deeper into the soil of God's marvelous love.

I believe grieving is a privilege. To grieve has meant you have loved. If you have loved, then you have truly sought God's heart.

My last visit with Jay was on a Thursday. He no longer was speaking. I was reading to him in-between suctioning his airway. At one point, our eyes met, and I believe this is what those eyes of his expressed: "It was on your God-given to-do list to come here today to show your love to me. I know you love me, and I will always love you!"

I have no doubt ... Just as Holy Scripture proclaims, Jay is born again ... and talking up a storm! I once knew a man called Bojangles and he talked to me!

~~~

Excerpts from the Eulogy of Reed Sevitts

As comedian Ron White has said, "I had the right to remain silent, but I did not have the ability."

I, too, have the right to remain silent, but because of Jay Jordan's inspiring friendship, "I do not have the ability."

Mitch Albom wrote a book titled, *Tuesdays with Morrie*, about his visits with an aging college professor who was dying and how that professor passed along valuable life lessons to the author.

Well, my Thursdays with Jay also revealed rich life lessons. Some of them are:

- Never feed an ALS patient Reuben sandwiches and beer the day after he has had a feeding tube surgically implanted.

- Do not induce laughter while irrigating a feeding tube.

- Never let an ALS patient drive a motorized wheelchair after holding [what we called[a "Kentucky Communion."

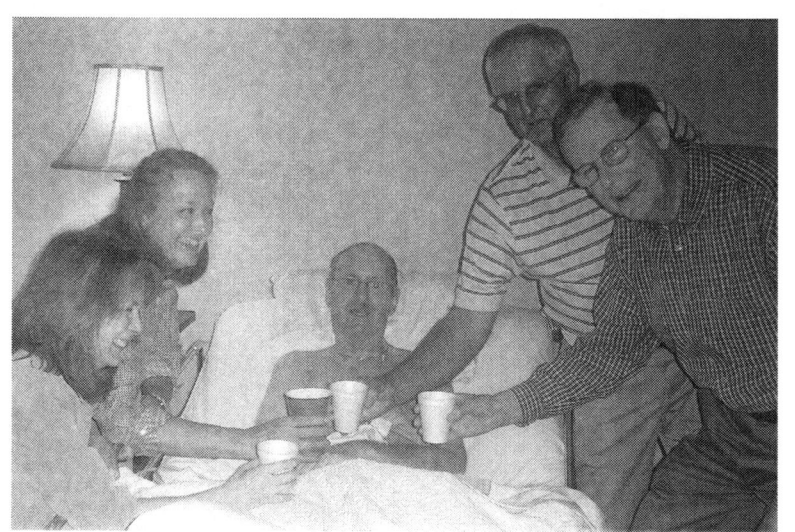

Celebrating communion the Kentucky way- with moonshine and grape juice.
L to r Ruth Gaines, Donna Sevitts, Reed Sevitts, and Rick Gaines

My Thursdays with Jay came about when his mobility had been decreasing rapidly. In Katie's desperation, she called for some assistance in the church bulletin. When the sign-up sheet came around, I immediately volunteered. My skeptical wife, Donna, reminded me that Katie was looking for people with medical training. But despite my lack of training, I felt a strong calling to sign up. I reasoned that Jay and Katie would screen out anyone that they felt could not handle the task.

They were very patient with me and slowly broke me into the tasks required, which multiplied as Jay's ALS progressed. Many of you have heard the saying that "If the Lord brings you to it, He will bring you through it." I stand before you today as a witness to this truth, and my time with Jay and Katie has made me a better person.

Matthew 13:31–32 states that the kingdom of Heaven is like a mustard seed, which a man took and planted in his field. Though it is the smallest of all seeds, it grows into the largest of the garden plants and becomes a tree, so the birds of the air come and perch on its branches.

Jay Jordan's faith was like an entire field of mustard seeds. Those of us privileged to serve him were allowed to perch on his branches of faith and receive a mustard seed of faith to grow within us.

He exhibited total dependence on God and always displayed a willingness to do His will. Jay's earthen body may have been broken and all of its contents spilled out, but the essence of Jay's faith has been absorbed into our hearts, and we'll carry him with us for the rest of our days.

I am confident Jay is in Heaven, in his new and perfect body with Jesus, who has an arm around him and is telling him, "Well done, good and faithful servant. You got through to them!"

~~~

Jay's chosen pallbearers were the friends who served him at his bedside: Charles Cox, David Jett, Larry Green, Rick Gaines, Alan Bailar, Reed Sevitts, Jim Meyer, Jeff Borchardt, and Scott Rowlett. Honorary pallbearers were Ted York and Gary Cairns (now deceased), who acted as liaison and coordinator between the Jordan family and the caring church members who came into our home and helped carry the mat.

Lunch that afternoon was served in our backyard, under a large tent. Jay would have appreciated all the stories that were as sumptuous and plentiful as the delicious food prepared by gracious hands. Marcia Niswonger and Donna Sevitts, "the Church Ladies," did their usual wonderful job of hospitality and service.

Later, I helped serve communion at our Saturday evening worship service at church. Pastor Mike Bowie prayed with me for God to grant strength for the forthcoming days. The Bailars returned to the house with the children and me. We laughed and toasted Jay and life.

A swirl of emotional highs and lows followed. For the first few days and weeks, I felt the proverbial weight had lifted from my shoulders, knowing that Jay was beyond his pain. The medical reminders—hospital bed, Hoyer lift, oxygen equipment, feeding tubes, wheelchairs—had been removed from our home. In the evenings, I'd sink into my easy chair before the large picture window that connected me with a view of the backyard, now green and in full bloom. Tipper would sink beside Jay's recliner, her eyes expressing bewilderment at the loss of her master and best friend.

"I know how you feel, girl," I whispered. After such a commotion with people bustling in and out, all of us fussing over Jay's care, the silence was deafening.

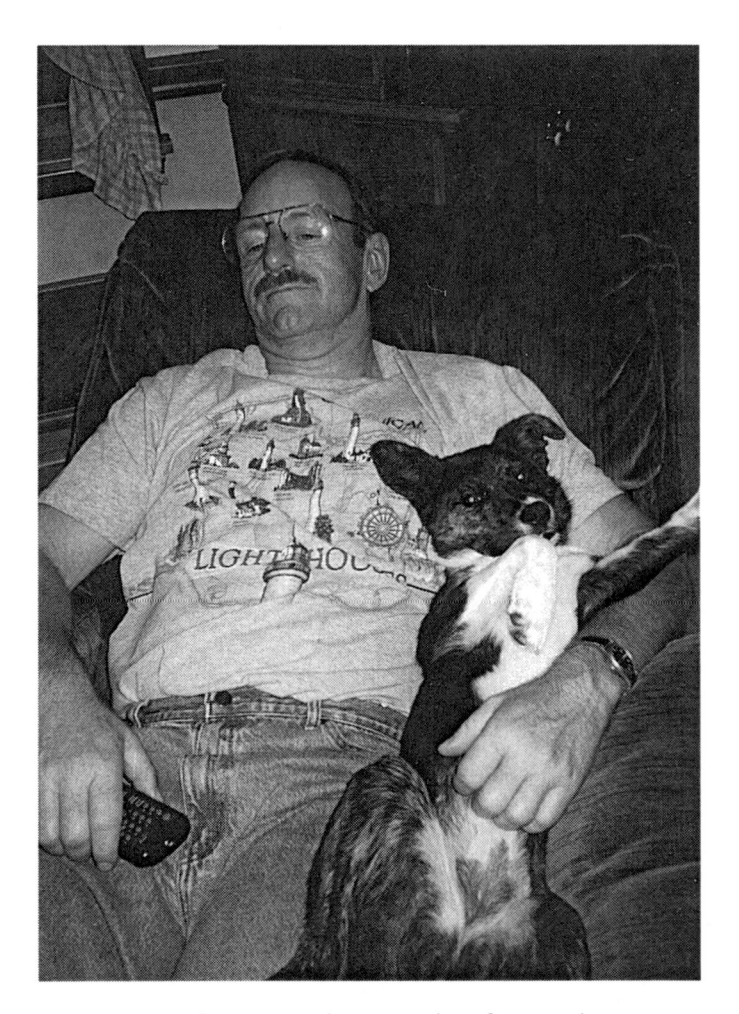

Jay and Tipper reclining in their favorite chair

Be still and know that I am God.
Psalm 46:10a

CHAPTER FIFTEEN

HOW MY GREATEST PAIN BECAME MY GREATEST PURPOSE

For me to live is Christ and to die is gain.—Philippians 1:21

Although I had great aspirations of being organized and purposeful after Jay's funeral, even finishing the smallest task proved to be impossible. In those first weeks, I would get mired in the details of hanging a curtain or sorting paperwork or sending an e-mail. I'd either forget to pay a bill altogether or pay it twice! Although there was plenty to keep me busy—settling Jay's estate, cleaning, reorganizing, sending notes of appreciation, starting a job search—I couldn't focus, as though lost in a fog.

As is common for most new widows and widowers, I quickly learned that socializing with couples friends now felt awkward. The discomfort with being single in social settings showed, as though my insecurities were under a bright spotlight. People didn't seem to know what to say. Nor did I.

I'm sure everyone was concerned. They would ask things like, "How are you?" That was a question I couldn't answer simply. Yet, it didn't seem appropriate to delve into details when encountering people at church or the grocery store.

There was no denying that a season of life had come to an end in more ways than one. When Jay died, all of my relationships were either altered or faded away entirely. I sensed that some people, whom I had grown to love like family, felt their job was finished. I wanted to tell most of our friends, "I don't know how to live yet without him—or without you." Thankfully, Alan and Pamela Bailar kept in frequent touch during those first months and helped me adjust.

I didn't seem to fit anywhere: in my church cell group (for couples) or even our home, especially since it had been built to accommodate Jay's special needs. Now that our home's primary purpose had been served, I didn't feel comfortable remaining there for the long term due to the reminders in every room, nook, and cranny. I might as well have been tumbleweed, rolling about in a windswept desert.

> *Lord, I've been grieving the loss of Jay for the final*
> *two-and-a-half years of his life.*
> *I want to move past the grief and LIVE!"*
> *All aspects of my life need to be redefined … but how?*

Unfortunately, grief takes its bittersweet time. There was no way to hurry the process along, and I had a long way to go.

> The Lord is close to the brokenhearted;
> He rescues those who are crushed in spirit.
> —Psalm 34:18

My coping mechanisms became engaging in yoga or swimming class with Pamela, and going out to lunch with friends. Also, during those first weeks and months alone, Luke and I flew to New York City to attend one of Matt's play productions. It was refreshing to go sightseeing with my sons in that exciting venue, where reminders of Jay and life's adjustments were far removed. Later, Sarah and I would explore the magic of San Francisco by cable car. We had all dealt with grief in our own separate ways over the course of Jay's illness. Now, we needed to make fresh memories and regroup as a family.

I had been so busy with Jay that now was the time to refocus on my adult children and applaud their personalities and inherent value. God in His wisdom knew how much our son, Luke, would mean to us (though I'm embarrassed and a little amused to admit that I'd wished for a girl back then). I saw Matt perform on stage and was again thankful for his special, loving personality and the unique way he bolstered my spirits during the toughest time our family had ever faced. And how many times had my elusive, impulsive Sarah whispered to me how special I was as her stepfather was dying? And who quietly asked my friends to take care of me?

During these visits, I realized I was capturing moments with them that Jay was missing. I hoped he could see us and share my pride in them and the way they were coping with their loss.

Thank you God, for our precious children.

Just six weeks after Jay's death, Pamela and I spent a week at the time-share property Jay and I had bought years ago in Hilton Head, South Carolina. Aside from hours spent strolling the beach, riding bikes, devouring a lot of ice cream, and exploring shops, we mapped out my dreams for this book based on journals and the scrapbooks following the course of Jay's journey with ALS.

In addition, our greeting card business was created to meet the emotional and spiritual needs of caregivers of the elderly and terminally ill. Pamela, a caregiver who had nursed her beloved stepfather during his losing battle with cancer, joined me in this quest to comfort the hearts of those carrying the mat.

We had long observed that messages inscribed inside standard greeting cards in today's market seemed trite for those facing death and dying. As a result, we launched Forever and Ever Cards, Incorporated. Luke used his photography skills to capture remarkable images exemplifying God's creative power and character as the front cover designs of our cards. We wrote the inscriptions inside to complement the photograph and theme. (Please refer to appendix 2 for more information and how to order Forever and Ever Cards).

> Now to Him who is able to do immeasurably more
> than all we ask or imagine,
> according to His power that is at work within us. Amen.
> —Ephesians 3:20

Already in those first few weeks, I had begun to miss Jay the way he was before his illness. I missed everything from his savvy computer skills to his perfect, stress-relieving neck massages. I found myself talking to him as though he were in the room with me. At times, when I'd do something thoughtless, like lose my credit cards or lock my keys in the trunk, I could imagine him rolling his eyes and cajoling me. When I tried to eat a meal alone, I imagined him sitting across the table and would talk with him about things that had happened that day or a concern.

How I loved being with people who had a special connection with Jay! For a while, we could talk openly and unashamedly about him. Remembering him kept him alive and whole, still a vital part of our lives. With the ring he betrothed still adorning my ring finger, I pondered how to press forward without him. All I could manage was one step at a time. Perhaps someday, I'd step out from under the overcast gloom of depression and into the sunshine of hope and renewed purpose.

Meanwhile, my friend Cheryl Jett advised, "Katie, embrace the memories with your arms open wide!"

One night, during a trip to Michigan with my mom and sister, the memories came so fast and furiously that I wanted to touch them and hold them and keep them … cocktail hour, when Jay and I would get lost in winding conversation that drew us close; long walks, exploring the woods for deer and whippoorwills; taking the kids to the beach; simple things, like feeding the ducks at a nearby lake … the laughter and fun of getting all dressed up to dine at a very casual restaurant, looking totally out of place!

Along with cherishing the memories comes that integral, haunting part of grief called guilt. *Had I encouraged him to exercise and keep active enough?*

Had I provided him access to books and the computer to keep his mind active? Maybe if I had been more patient ... Those and many more regrets and concerns kept unfurling as the weeks and months rolled on.

My one comfort in this regard was something Jay had said a couple of months before he died: "I don't want anyone feeling guilty or thinking they didn't do enough when I was alive. I don't need anyone going down that road. It doesn't accomplish a darn thing."

After my season of trips subsided, I faced myriad decisions, including the following:

- Should I resume my career yet?

- Should I sell the house and relocate?

- If so, where should I move?

- Should I seek doctor's advice about feelings of depression and lack of self-worth?

Once again, writing in my journal seemed to be a comforting lifeline to God and a way to work through the decision-making process. In fact, journaling was a safe way to deposit all confusion about the past, present, and future. Slowly but surely, I began to leave concerns in the Lord's capable, loving hands.

As I began praying for God to make His guidance known, I sensed His personal word meant for me: "I will never leave you nor forsake you." Then, a peace that passes all understanding washed over me.

Lord, with support from friends, and love from you,
keep me focused forward and not back.
Help me let go of guilt and forgive and love myself.
The doctor says I should go back to work.
Friends advise me to take some time off.
I feel the need to reboot, shut down, and simply listen to You.
Lord ... Slow me down.
Help me "just be" and focus on you.

Clear my mind of all the useless clutter.
Only then will my path become clear.
In Your precious Name,
Amen.

When Bobette died on August 30, 2007, following a fall, I was asked to deliver her eulogy. What an honor to speak from my heart about a truly genuine friend and woman of God. I thought of Jay and Bobette's joyful friendship reunion in Heaven, just as they had planned over pizza at our house two years before.

Later, as we departed the cemetery following Bobette's graveside remembrances, Luke and I decided to visit Jay's grave. Our son had never asked for much during his dad's illness, but as we approached the grave, Luke asked if his favorite Scripture could be added to Jay's headstone:

> For me to live is Christ and to die is gain.
> —Philippians 1:21

My mind backtracked to another day, when Jay and I stood with other parents on the football field of our son's high school, awaiting Luke's moment of glory to be announced during the fall sports halftime program. As the announcer called his name and referenced our son's achievements, Jay and I walked from our position toward the fifty-yard line. There was Luke, presenting us with two yellow roses. Over the loud speakers, we learned that Luke's favorite Bible verse was Philippians 1:21.

This had become the Scripture Jay and I claimed for the two-and-a-half years we struggled with ALS ... the verse that was printed in Jay's funeral service program. Luke's request to add the verse to his father's stone was perfect.

Luke encouraged me to read the two verses that follow Philippians 1:21 when I got home. This is how the entire passage reads:

> For me to live is Christ and to die is gain.

If I am to go on living in the body, this
will mean fruitful labor for me.
Yet what shall I choose? I do not know.
I am torn between the two.
I desire to depart and to be with Christ, which is better by far.

Through our son, I was reminded that Jay had the better option. What wonderful reassurance that his spirit was with the Lord—alive and well! And now, these verses are my peace, as I continue to live for Christ.

In coping with grief, God began showing me truth after truth. Slowly, healing began to take place, as my awareness grew to encompass the pain of others who were losing or had lost their spouses. The focus began to move away from what I suffered to what I could do to have a positive impact on others' lives. Beyond grief, a fulfilling ministry of encouragement was taking shape.

One night, I attended a worship service held in a small storefront church with my friend Ruth Gaines, who has since passed away. The worship leader delivered a powerful testimony about her husband's seven years of physical suffering and painful death. Afterward, the three of us prayed and wept together, because we could intimately identify with each other through our grief experiences. She stressed the importance of accepting Jesus as Lord over everything, not just parts of our lives.

I needed to hear from someone who has been where I am,
that the hurt will continue as will the tears.
Lord, how important it is to have instrumental people near
who will say nothing until You direct them to be there
with a physical presence, a touch, or a hug. That's so powerful.
Diane said tonight that
she doesn't believe our husbands' deaths were in Your plan or purpose ...
but it is up to us to make their lives have a purpose
by how we react and carry forward.
Thank you for these authentic women
who cried and shared their hearts with me tonight, Lord.

God continued to thread together the pieces of my broken heart through one experience after another. One day, I was on the treadmill, reading about overcoming adversity in the popular Bible study book, *Experiencing God* by Henry Blackaby. I began to understand that God has had me in a "desert experience" for a purpose. He has been quiet, because I needed that time for reflection, not action. I hadn't been ready to move forward. Until now.

Suddenly I felt like I heard God loud and clear:
"Get busy on that book. You have a story to tell!"

Soon after that, Pastor Mike Bowie's lesson in Bible study was about an attitude of gratitude. He repeatedly called on me, so he must have zoned in on my struggle to find my bearings beyond losing Jay. He pointed out that God knew I could be "trusted with trial," because I would use it for His greater purpose. It became clear God's intent was never to tear me down but to build me up. I had a hope and a future in Him.

Before I left, Mike sat down with me. A visionary with great compassion, Mike assured me he could see great strength in my soul. "Out of the tragedy of Jay's death," he said, "a ministry will come."

One of my classmates approached to thank me for a particular time I had talked with her at a Recovery Service. She had been looking for me ever since, to thank me, she said. The knowledge that God's grace had touched her life through me was like finding a little piece of Heaven! We prayed together in a spirit of thanksgiving.

Although losing couples friends after Jay's death pierced my heart, I began to realize that not everyone could be expected to go the distance with me. Some were called to be in our lives for the season Jay and I needed them most. As I began to search deeper to find God's purpose for my life, I realized His supply of friendships for me was abundantly gracious. It became well with my soul to release the unresolved pain I had been harboring.

Releasing my hurt to God has brought closure. Through God's grace, knowing He provides for every need, I began to let go of the anger, the confusion, the sense of abandonment. I am still learning to let go. At the resolution of this process is peace.

God places the right people in your life at the right time.
Only by letting go of my fear of abandonment can I let God.
God, I hear you. I thank you. I praise you.
I will keep an attitude of gratitude—
For my family, my faith, and my finances.
But Lord thank you for my friends—those you gave us for a season
and those who are willing to go the distance in this healing process.
Amen.

Another assignment in the "Experiencing God" study was to concentrate on my love relationship with the Father. I couldn't think of a better place to listen to God than in nature. Since it was a beautiful, autumn afternoon, I took my book and a blanket to sit upon, and headed out to the cemetery. As had been my habit for such a long time, I read to Jay, as though he could still hear me.

Autumn's golden glow conjured memories, as I watched the leaves that seemed to "cheer" in the wind as they waved from the branches overhead. I remembered walking with Jay and the boys through the woods to collect autumn leaves, riding bikes with Jay, feeding the ducks, boating, traveling together. God was showing me I had stored a treasury of memories in my heart, and the key to unlocking them was drawing away for time to be with Him in a quiet place like this.

God began to speak to me about my concerns about being widowed. Still fairly young, I worried about being alone for so many years. How bittersweet to realize no one could possibly love me more than Jay. Wondering whether I would marry again or what my future looked like had troubled me to no end. There, in that quiet place, the assurance came:

Even if I am never to have another earthly relationship,
I will be okay.
God is my Friend, Father, Husband, Brother.
He is enough.

I watched the leaves sprinkle down onto the blanket where I sat and thought of the first book Jay had ever read to me: *The Fall of Freddie the Leaf,* by Leo Buscaglia. It is a beloved story about life and death, written for children of all ages, even Jay and me.

He had loved to read to me about Freddie the Leaf that does not want to let go in the autumn of the year. He fears the coming of winter and wonders what will happen to him. He wonders what will happen to his friends, the leaves who hang precariously on the tree branch with him, waiting for the wind to sweep them away. He thinks he can prevent the inevitable. In the end, he falls and realizes he feels comfortable and sleepy, lying still in the snow. What Freddie doesn't know is that in spring, the snow will melt and he—Freddie—will blend with the melted snow to help nourish the ground for new life to sprout.

God had been wrapping me in such peaceful, healing thoughts that I hadn't realized forty-five minutes had zipped by! When I left, I felt warm and relaxed. I no longer felt anxious and isolated, but protected and loved.

I have decided I must no longer live in the past, wondering what might have been. I must look for what will be. He makes all things new. I get up every morning and make a conscious choice to move forward. If I am true to staying the course, God will show me what is next in store.

Since Jay's death on June 27, 2007, he has missed so much. Our little granddaughter, Selah Grace, was born to Luke and Elizabeth on January 15, 2010. Her big brother, Ethan, is now five years old and loves to come play with his Grammie Katie. Levi Kristopher entered this life during an unexpected home birth on December 13, 2011.

When I babysat for Selah recently, Luke and Elizabeth took their little son to visit his grandpa Jay's grave. Ethan spoke of Jay like he's known him all of his little life. (I wouldn't be surprised if he visits Ethan, for Ethan embodies his exuberance for life!)

Sarah graduated from nursing school. She now has her dream job as an emergency room RN is San Francisco. Matt is a married man now. I have completed my third year at Edison Community College as a faculty member in the physical therapist assisting program.

In April 2010, I sold our house and moved to a smaller, more manageable one in our community of Troy, Ohio. I continue to have a small support group, fondly referred to as God's Girls, of those who gave up their evenings for fifteen months to get Jay ready for bed.

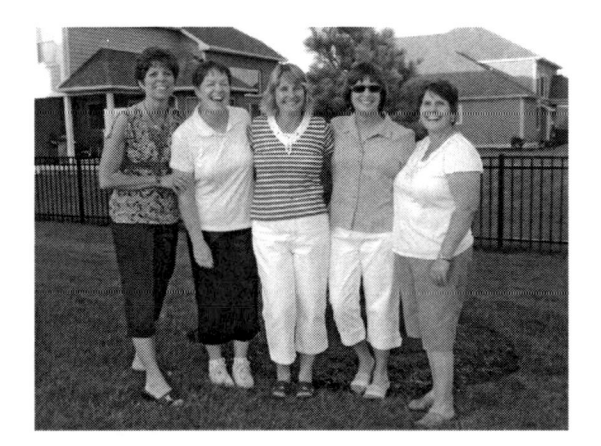

God's Girls celebrate Jay's first eternal birthday . From l to r: Deb Meyer, Kathy Conrad, Beth Thoele, me, Pamela Bailar.

Best of all, the promised book Jay so wanted me to write has been written. It honors a life well lived and validates a community of caregivers who helped me carry Jay's mat to the feet of his Savior. Until I join him, I will keep my promise to share our story and be an advocate for caregivers wherever I go.

Our greatest pain can become our greatest purpose.

APPENDIX 1

CAREGIVING ONLINE RESOURCES

CaringBridge www.caringbridge.org

> A nonprofit web service connecting family and friends during a critical illness and treatment. Patients and caregivers can draw strength from messages of support.

Family Caregiving 101 www.familycaregiving101.org

> The National Family Caregivers Association (NFCA) and the National Alliance for Caregiving (NAC)—leaders in the movement to better understand and assist family caregivers—have joined together to recognize, support and advise this vital group of Americans. Family caregivers have been part of America's health care picture for a very long time. Yet, their roles and special needs are just being acknowledged.

> More than 50 million family caregivers in this country provide care for a chronically ill or aging family member or friend. It is estimated that family caregivers provide some $306 million in services to America's overburdened health care system.

> Our outreach program is called "Family Caregiving: It's Not All Up to You." This effort is national in scope, and includes radio announcements and magazine and newspaper advertisements that connect family caregivers to information and services that can help improve their lives and the level of care they can offer their loved ones. Research has shown that millions of Americans are taking on the burden of caregiving

without acknowledging the effect it has on their lives, and without realizing there is relief out there for them.

The centerpiece of the "Family Caregiving: It's Not All Up to You" campaign is familycaregiving101.org. The site is designed to provide caregivers with the basic tools, skills and information they need to protect their own physical and mental health while they provide high quality care for their loved one. It is also a place for family caregivers to return again and again as new levels of caregiving are reached. Advertising messages, crafted with the assistance of family caregivers themselves, assure caregivers across America that they are not alone, and encourage caregivers to take better care of themselves and their loved one by visiting the site and asking for help.

National Alliance for Caregiving www.caregiving.org

Established in 1996, the National Alliance for Caregiving is a non-profit coalition of national organizations focusing on issues of family caregiving. Alliance members include grassroots organizations, professional associations, service organizations, disease-specific organizations, a government agency, and corporations ... Recognizing that family caregivers provide important societal and financial contributions toward maintaining the well-being of those they care for, the Alliance's mission is to be the objective national resource on family caregiving with the goal of improving the quality of life for families and care recipients.

National Family Caregivers Association www.nfcacares.org

The National Family Caregivers Association educates, supports, empowers and speaks up for the more than 65 million Americans who care for loved ones with a chronic illness or disability or the frailties of old age. NFCA reaches across the boundaries of diagnoses, relationships and life stages to help transform family caregivers' lives by removing barriers to health and well being.

NFCA's core Caring Every Day messages are:

Believe in Yourself.
Protect Your Health.
Reach Out for Help.
Speak Up for Your Rights.

APPENDIX 2

FOREVER AND EVER CARDS, INC.

Katie Jordan and Pamela Bailar

Forever and Ever, Inc. (www.foreverandevercards.com), is a niche greeting card company that grew out of experience as caregivers of loved ones diagnosed with ALS and cancer. Forever and Ever, Inc., specializes in cards appropriate to send to the caregivers, family, and friends of persons who are seriously or terminally ill. Though the passion is for this particular market, the cards are also suitable for anyone needing hope, encouragement, and a sense of community.

Understanding that it is incredibly difficult to find the right sentiment in a standard card, Forever and Ever, Inc., fills this void. The cards are uniquely designed to resonate with caregivers' spirit. Cards feature a distinctive, short sentiment, varnished picture front, and colored border. A framed card instantly becomes an inspirational artwork.

APPENDIX 3

HELPFUL HINTS ON HOME MODIFICATION

*Published by the Central and Southern
Ohio Chapter of ALS Newsletter*
by Katie and Jay Jordan

Jay and I began our journey with ALS in January of 2005. Even though we had our suspicions in the fall, we kept an open mind and heart to the other possibilities.

At the time, our son, Luke, was in his senior year of high school, and we had been making future plans of downsizing. We lived in a two-story home. Our bedroom and full bath were on the second floor. There was also a step-down family room and sunroom, and Jay's office was in the basement.

As Jay's symptoms progressed, we made accommodations, including moving his office to the first-floor dining room. Additionally, we installed a large step with a landing in our garage that accommodated a walker. Jay navigated the flight of stairs to and from the second floor once in the morning and once at night, with someone accompanying him.

In the spring, we began to look seriously for a ranch-style home, or a home that had the master bedroom and bath on the first floor. We continued to be forward-thinking and looked for a house that would accommodate a wheelchair and allow modifications to the bathroom. Nothing was on the market that addressed these needs. We made the decision to build in the spring.

Building in itself is a journey, which was a learning experience for us and the builder. We would like to share the good and the bad with you, if you are either seeking to build or modify your existing home.

- Meet with more than one builder. Ask them how many handicapped-accessible homes they have built, and ask to see their work.

- Insist that all communication during the process be in writing.

- House plans should be viewed in three dimensions. We found it very hard to visualize area size and fit without three-dimensional imaging. This may not apply if you are accustomed to reading blueprints.

- Persons with disabilities need to have access to the house at all times from the beginning of the process. This could be a simple plywood path or as elaborate as poured concrete. Not being able to see the house as it is progressing is not conducive to a smooth building and communication process. After all, you are the one who will need to determine the position of switches, walls, and doorways, as well as any other modifications you deem necessary. Remember that your home needs to fit your specific needs.

- The three most important rooms to us became the bathroom, bedroom, and kitchen. These rooms need to be large enough to accommodate you and at least one caregiver, as well as additional equipment that comes with the progression of the disease (hospital bed, shower chairs, Hoyer lifts, BiPAP machines, etc.).

- All entrances and exits from your home should be flat or

have a minimum elevation. Anywhere in your house where there is a step will eventually become an eliminated access area for the patient.

- A safe room should be incorporated into all plans. Someone confined to a wheelchair will be unable to access a basement or crawl space should inclement weather, such as a tornado, occurs.

- The garage needs to be wider and deeper than the standard size to allow access to and from the vehicle without having to go outside.

After living in our house for eight months, we learned many things we could have done differently that would have saved us extra work, frustration, and expense:

- Do not accept minimum ADA standards.

- The area that is most questionable is the bathroom. As strength in an ALS patient diminishes, getting on and off the commode becomes a major issue. The commode height should be predicated on the size of the individual. We found the ADA minimum standard was inadequate for our needs.

- The commode needs to be several feet from the wall on both sides to allow for wheelchair mobility as well as caregiver access from either side to assist with transfers. There are grab bars available that attach to the wall and fold up out of the way for easier access.

- Grab bars should be mounted both inside and outside the shower. The shower should contain a fixed or drop-down seat.

- Bathroom code only requires one electrical outlet by each sink. This number was inadequate for our needs. Two additional electrical outlets were installed for a wall heater and bidet, which we mounted on our commode for personal hygiene.

- Have pocket doors placed on all bathrooms.

- The bathroom sink has to be high enough and shaped so a wheelchair can maneuver under it. The faucet controls on the sink should have eight-inch holes instead of four-inch holes.

- Consider putting hardwood, tile, or vinyl in the bedroom and bathroom instead of carpet. Pushing heavy equipment such as a Hoyer lift, wheelchair, or shower chair is too difficult. Cleanup from spills is also easier with a hard surface. Keeping the carpet clean is more difficult no matter how low the pile.

- Table heights should accommodate your wheelchair. Call the wheelchair vendor to find the clearance you need to easily fit under all surfaces.

- Test all light fixture placements from your wheelchair. As muscles weaken, it is difficult to reach a normally placed switch. A few inches make a big difference.

- Most doorways require a 90-degree turn. Even with wider hallways, this is a difficult turn for the most experienced wheelchair operator. Doors should be placed at a 45-degree angle.

- Have wheelchair access onto and off your property. Most driveways have a significant lip onto the street. Talk to the builder and concrete contractor, and request a wheelchair-accessible ramp onto the street.

CPSIA information can be obtained at www.ICGtesting.com
Printed in the USA
BVOW071703010612

291583BV00001B/2/P

9 781449 749552